Praise for

HEAL
YOUR
MIND

"*Heal Your Mind* is a much-needed guidebook to
understanding the relationship between your mind and
your health. It is a treasure chest of insights that merge wisdom
and essential health information. And, it's a great read."

— **Caroline Myss**, *New York Times* best-selling
author of *Anatomy of the Spirit* and *Defy Gravity*

"Holism, as detailed in this wonderful text, represents
an empowering platform from which we can truly embrace
the underpinnings of our motivations, emotions, and
perceptions of the world around us. *Heal Your Mind*'s expansive,
far-reaching, and unrestrained perspective compassionately
guides the reader with an actionable plan that will immediately
help you reframe your sense of what it means to be at peace."

— **David Perlmutter, M.D.**, *New York Times* best-selling
author of *Grain Brain* and *Brain Maker*

"As a psychiatrist, I am thrilled when a book that can
heal the mind becomes available. In their brilliant new work,
Mona Lisa Schulz and Louise Hay blend their wisdom and
expertise to offer profound healing advice for both mind and
body. This book is truly a treasure, combining elements of
modern brain chemistry and nutrition with intuitional insight
and affirmations that can help to rewire and restore brain
function. I highly recommend *Heal Your Mind*."

— **Brian L. Weiss, M.D.**, *New York Times* best-selling
author of *Many Lives, Many Masters*

HEAL

YOUR

MIND

For Children

The Adventures of Lulu

I Think, I Am! (with Kristina Tracy)

Lulu and the Ant: A Message of Love

Lulu and the Dark: Conquering Fears

Lulu and Willy the Duck:
Learning Mirror Work

Audio Programs

Anger Releasing

Cancer

Change and Transition

Dissolving Barriers

Embracing Change

The Empowering Women Gift Collection

Feeling Fine Affirmations

Forgiveness/Loving the Inner Child

How to Love Yourself

Meditations for Personal Healing

Meditations to Heal Your Life
(audio book)

Morning and Evening Meditations

101 Power Thoughts

Overcoming Fears

The Power Is Within You (audio book)

The Power of Your Spoken Word

Receiving Prosperity

Self-Esteem Affirmations (subliminal)

Self-Healing

Stress-Free (subliminal)

Totality of Possibilities

What I Believe and Deep Relaxation

You Can Heal Your Life (audio book)

You Can Heal Your Life Study Course

Your Thoughts Create Your Life

DVDs

Dissolving Barriers

Receiving Prosperity

You Can Heal Your Life Study Course

You Can Heal Your Life, The Movie
(also available in an expanded edition)

Card Decks

Healthy Body Cards

I Can Do It® Cards

I Can Do It® Cards . . . for Creativity,
Forgiveness, Health, Job Success,
Wealth, Romance

Power Thought Cards

Power Thoughts for Teens

Power Thought Sticky Cards

Wisdom Cards

Calendar

I Can Do It® Calendar
(for each individual year)

*Available from Hay House
Please visit:

Hay House USA: www.hayhouse.com®
Hay House Australia: www.hayhouse.com.au
Hay House UK: www.hayhouse.co.uk
Hay House South Africa: www.hayhouse.co.za
Hay House India: www.hayhouse.co.in

○ ○ ○

HEAL YOUR MIND

Your PRESCRIPTION for WHOLENESS through MEDICINE, AFFIRMATIONS, and INTUITION

MONA LISA SCHULZ,
M.D., PH.D.,
with LOUISE HAY

HAY HOUSE, INC.
Carlsbad, California • New York City
London • Sydney • Johannesburg
Vancouver • New Delhi

Published and distributed in the United States by: Hay House, Inc.: www
.hayhouse.com® • *Published and distributed in Australia by:* Hay House
Australia Pty. Ltd.: www.hayhouse.com.au • *Published and distributed in
the United Kingdom by:* Hay House UK, Ltd.: www.hayhouse.co.uk • *Pub-
lished and distributed in the Republic of South Africa by:* Hay House
SA (Pty), Ltd.: www.hayhouse.co.za • *Distributed in Canada by:* Raincoast
Books: www.raincoast.com • *Published in India by:* Hay House Publishers
India: www.hayhouse.co.in

Indexer: Jay Kreider
Cover design: Michelle Polizzi • *Interior design:* Tricia Breidenthal

Note: The case studies found in this book are composites drawn from years of
clinical work. These are true to the spirit of the teaching and the treatment pro-
vided, although not to the experience of any one particular person.

Library of Congress Cataloging-in-Publication Data for the original edition:

Names: Schulz, Mona Lisa, author. | Hay, Louise L., author.
Title: Heal your mind : your prescription for wholeness through medicine,
    affirmations, and intuition / Mona Lisa Schulz, M.D., Ph.D., with Louise
    Hay.
Description: Carlsbad, California : Hay House, Inc., [2016]
Identifiers: LCCN 2016028067 | ISBN 9781401945145 (hardback)
Subjects: LCSH: Mental healing. | Mind and body. | Nervous
    system--Diseases--Treatment. | BISAC: BODY, MIND & SPIRIT / Healing /
    General. | HEALTH & FITNESS / Healing. | PSYCHOLOGY / Mental Health.
Classification: LCC RZ400 .S48 2016 | DDC 615.8/528--dc23 LC record available
    at https://lccn.loc.gov/2016028067

Tradepaper ISBN: 978-1-4019-4515-2

10 9 8 7 6 5 4 3 2 1
1st edition, October 2016
2nd edition, October 2017

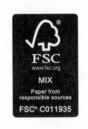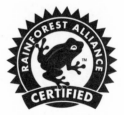

Printed in the United States of America

This is dedicated to
our wonderful minds.

LOVE THE MIND
YOU'RE WITH!

CONTENTS

A NOTE FROM LOUISE

Mona Lisa Schulz, whom I love and adore, promised me for ages that she would pull together scientific evidence to support what I'd been teaching for years. While I personally do not need proof to know that these methods work—I rely on what I call my "Inner Ding" to evaluate things—I know there are many people who will only consider a new idea if there is science behind it.

In our book *All Is Well: Heal Your Body with Medicine, Affirmations, and Intuition*, we presented the science and gave you a step-by-step way of moving from illness to wellness. In the process, I learned even more about my own work. I gained a much deeper understanding of what I'd been teaching all along, and I came to see even more vividly how interconnected our emotions, thoughts, and health really are.

This new book adds another dimension: it does for the mind what the first book did for the body, outlining the connections between emotional wellness and prescriptions for healing. I know you will use the information in this book to create a healthy and happy life.

INTRODUCTION

For my whole life, I have tried to run with the herd, to pass for normal. Like many women, I've tried to keep it together and maintain my mood on an even keel. When it comes to nerves, I haven't wanted to lose my nerve when "nerve" meant needing to be courageous, but I haven't wanted to become a bundle of nerves when I needed to be cool and collected. When it comes to focus, when taking an exam or even listening to a lecture, I've needed to focus and pay attention—but we're also told to meditate and become expanded and spacious in our awareness rather than narrowly focused. And then, finally, as I get older, I just don't want to "lose it." That doesn't mean avoiding emotional outbursts. That means I want to maintain my wits, keep my memory, keep a sharp mind. And yet even that's not enough. I want more. I want to be spiritual, intuitive, attuned, empathic. Is it possible to do all this and be healthy? Yes, it is.

But not everybody can have it all. Everybody has something different about them. You may have a gene in your family that predisposes toward depression or anxiety. You may have been diagnosed with ADHD, or you may have memory or brain fog, or something may have happened in your life such as trauma or abuse, or you may have witnessed tragedy, which may have made you more likely to have depression, anxiety, or memory problems. You can heal your mind, acquire wholeness, with medicine, affirmations, and intuition. How? I'm going to show you, because I've spent my whole life trying to do it.

We're all born with a challenge here or there. We have trouble handling a problem. We go to school to figure out how to help somebody else with that problem. In my case, I had two brain disorders—narcolepsy and epilepsy—both of which helped me with my career in intuition. And I would assume that those two disorders have increased my risk for other health problems that have affected my mood, made me at times a bundle of nerves, and made it hard for me to focus and pay attention. So what did I do? I went to school. I went to school *a lot*. One of my mottoes is "Nothing succeeds like excess." So, when other people were fitting in, being cool and collected (but mostly cool), I wasn't. I was on the sidelines with a book, with a pen—this was before tablets and iPhones—and I was reading, reading, reading. Getting my B.A. from Brown, my M.D., and my Ph.D., ultimately becoming a neuroanatomist and a board-certified psychiatrist with a specialty in neuropsychiatry. In the course of all that, I learned that you couldn't figure out everything with intellect alone, and I learned I had a facility for medical intuition: the capacity to understand how certain sensations in our body, certain illnesses, let us know when something in our life is out of balance. More on that later.

Suffice it to say, I have spent over 20 years on my education, not including high school. I pursued higher education from 1978 to 1998 in order to teach you, ultimately, how to heal your mind in pursuit of becoming whole. You can learn along with me how to do this.

WHOLENESS IN MIND

For centuries, scientists, psychologists, and spiritual teachers have tried to unravel why we suffer emotionally. There are a lot of facts. There are a lot of citations. We know that melancholy, sadness, crisis, and trauma do become wired in the brain and the body. Today, medicine has had to come to grips with the idea that every illness can be made worse or better by our emotional state.

Louise Hay and I have been talking about these connections for decades. Louise's first book, *Heal Your Body: The Mental Causes of Physical Illness*, first published in 1984, is a groundbreaking book in this area. In her tome (actually a tiny little blue book), she claims that the good and the dis-ease in our life are the results of thoughts, that thoughts form our experience. This is interesting because now, in the 21st century, we understand that our brains reshape themselves through plasticity throughout our life. We are affected by our thoughts and our feelings, for good or for ill. Louise, over the decades of her career, has helped people change their thoughts and their experiences with affirmations to help them improve their health; now medicine and science are doing the same through cognitive behavioral therapy and dialectical behavioral therapy, stress reduction, and "mindfulness" therapy. Louise could have gotten a co-pay!

For over 30 years, I have worked in the field of medical intuition. Knowing only a client's name and age over the phone, I describe how a specific emotional pattern in their life aggravates certain organs in their body. I teach the client how to name the emotional pattern, respond to it effectively, and then release it; I also explain how if they don't, the emotion and feeling can become more entrenched in the form of a physical problem in their body. To help facilitate the process, I teach them how an array of solutions can help support their body, whether it's medicines, herbs, nutritional supplements, affirmations, or a variety of other suggestions to support their healing process. Whether it's the brain or the body, to become whole, we all need nutritional supplements, herbs, conventional medicine, sometimes surgery, affirmations, and a variety of body work, from acupuncture to chiropractic. It's important that you, the consumer, know everything that's available in front of you like a buffet. A plethora of solutions. A cornucopia of remedies from which you and your practitioner may choose to create whole health.

Back when I was trying to finish my B.A. at Brown, I was falling all over the place with my neurological problem, I was falling asleep. It's very hard to learn when you're asleep, mind you. Ultimately, they gave me a medicine, an anticonvulsant, during my last year at Brown, and it woke me up. This medicine changed my life. I went from the 2.22 average I'd had for five years to a 4.0. I had my *Flowers for Algernon* moment. However, once I graduated, two weeks later I went running (something I used to do to stay awake), and I ran across a bridge. Who knows what happened? Maybe I fell asleep, maybe I had a seizure; all I know is, I never saw the truck. The truck hit me and threw me 86 feet. I had four fractures in my pelvis, several broken ribs, a collapsed lung, and a shattered scapula. I won't bore you with the details. Suffice it to say, I was in the ICU for 4 days, in the hospital for 11. But afterward, none the worse for wear, I did an awful lot of things to heal, as I had done for my brain disorder. I used everything I could find to put myself back into a whole state. I did acupuncture. I used Chinese herbs. I did craniosacral therapy. I did osteopathy. And three months later, I ran a 10K and I won it in 5.5-minute miles, partly because it hurt so bad and I kept trying to outrun the pain. It felt cool to be able to do that, but I had to get off of the medicine because I was having a life-threatening side effect. So there I was, back to square one, and I didn't like losing my intellect, because that's what happened to the character in *Flowers for Algernon*: he has a treatment to make him smart, to cognitively challenge him, but at the end of the novel, it's reversed and he loses his intellect. It's as if the shade is pulled down on his mind. That is what happened to me. They tried a series of medicines—Dilantin, Mysoline—but none of them worked, and my doctor said, "You learned to live like this before. You can learn to live like this again."

It was very upsetting, to say the least. I tried a lot of things to find a solution, starting with a macrobiotic diet. At that point, medicine was not available, or I would have used it. I was living in this house with these other people who were a little on the depressed side, so I didn't want to spend a lot of time at home. Instead, I would go to bookstores, these wonderful little bookstores where they had crystals and so on. I walked into a bookstore on Newbury Street in Boston called Trident Booksellers, and I leaned against a shelf, and this little blue book fell off: *Heal Your Body*, by Louise Hay. And there were these things called affirmations, and she said that if you say them over again, you can change thought patterns that can make your health worse, while the new thought patterns made you better. If you want to follow along, the chart from *Heal Your Body* that connects specific thoughts to health problems and affirmations is in Appendix B.

You know how in the gym, you do reps with weights? I figured I would do reps with the affirmations. So one of the reps was "I love myself just the way I am." I would write that five times a day. "I love myself just the way I am. I love myself just the way I am. I love myself just the way I am. I love myself just the way I am. I love myself just the way I am." I got a journal, and I began doing the affirmations. And within three or four months, I woke up. I slowly learned various things that made my spells worse or made them better. I managed to slowly wake up, using the affirmations along with a macrobiotic diet and herbs.

Everybody has a story. If you're reading this book, you've had health problems, and you've tried to find solutions. You've tried medicines. You've tried herbs. You've tried nutritional supplements. You've tried a variety of things. You may also have depression. You may have anxiety. You may have problems with attention. You may have memory problems, addiction. You may have elements of your personality that need a little bit of smoothing—don't we all? And I'm going to help you learn how to heal your mind, which will ultimately heal your body, problem by problem, area of the brain by area of the brain. I'm going to teach you how to create wholeness. That's what this book is all about.

MEDICAL INTUITION AND THE MIND–BODY NETWORK

For centuries, we've talked about a network called the chakra system. In the terms of medical intuition, there are emotional centers. Why do I use this term? Because I'm an anatomist and a physician, and brain anatomy suggests that emotions are wired between the brain and the body. You'll go to some medical intuitives to talk about energy centers; I talk about emotional centers, but I also include energy. Each center, whatever you want to call it, corresponds to an area of your physical anatomy. Each center has a life situation and an emotion that affects an area of the body. This is the map that's going to help you create health. Yes, it is.

There are seven regions in this emotional/energy center system. Get yourself a piece of paper and write them down. While you're reading this book, circle the areas you have problems with. Why? Because you're going to be doing your first medical intuitive reading on yourself. You may want to use the chart in Appendix A as a guide.

These are the seven regions:

1. First center: bones, blood, immune system, skin, joints, and muscle. This physical region is affected by the health of our family or other groups of people.

2. Second center: reproductive organs like uterus, ovaries, vagina, prostate, testes, lower back, hips, and bladder. This area is associated with concerns about love and money.

3. Third center: digestive tract—esophagus, stomach, liver, gallbladder, colon, rectum, metabolism, pancreas, body image. This area is influenced by self-esteem, work, feeling good enough.

4. Fourth center: heart, breast, lungs. This region has to do with health, nurturance, and partnerships.

5. Fifth center: neck, thyroid, mouth, teeth, jaw. This area is influenced by our communication style and our healthy capacity to handle timing.

6. Sixth center: head, eyes, ears, brain. This area relates to perception, thought, and basic mental health.

7. Seventh center: life-threatening illnesses, or events in our lives that bring us to our knees. Not a discrete area of the physical body but affecting many parts of

the body, this region has to do with spirituality and
life purpose.

As you make a note of the areas where you have problems,
you're doing your own medical intuitive reading. By noting which
area of the body you have most of your problems in, you will
begin to know where most of your emotions are patterned.

What is medical intuition? In medical intuition, certain areas
of your body let you know when emotion has built up in a certain
area of your life. Certain organs in your body intuitively will let
you know that something that's emotionally bothering you needs
to change. So, if it's depression about a family member, anger
about a relative, anger about a mate, frustration about money, or
anxiety about work, and so on and so on, certain areas of your
body will murmur, nudge, or scream loudly when that area of
your emotional life needs to change.

Medical intuition lets us look at the function of the brain
alongside these seven centers as part of the larger mind-body
network. So your right brain is made up half of your emotions
and half of your intuition. Your left brain is for language, that is,
putting your feelings and intuition into words and action. So, for
health, if you can't take your feelings from the right brain, name
them, respond effectively, and release them, your health is going
to let you know medical-intuitively. Your right brain emotion and
intuition will travel down to your body, into one or more of those
seven centers, and talk to you through symptoms of disease.

HOW EMOTION TRANSLATES TO THE BODY

So, now you know that your body will tell you, through symptoms of health, when areas in your family, relationship, money,
and work are going great. Or, intuitively, your body will let you
know through health problems that those areas in your life aren't
going great. You can learn how to listen to the beginnings of your
feelings in your right brain, the area for intuition; how to detect

the beginning of sadness before it turns to depression. The beginning of fear before it turns to panic and anxiety. The beginning of anger before it turns to frustration and meltdown. Before these emotions affect your health, your attention, and ultimately other areas of your brain.

So let's do a hypothetical reading (or maybe not so hypothetical, since these issues are so common to all of us):

- Look at the areas on *your* reading: did you circle the first center, for problems such as immune disorders like allergies or infections? If you did, then ask yourself, *What's my family like? Do I have a lot of friends? Do I feel safe and secure in the world?*

- Or did you circle the second center areas—lower back, uterus, ovaries, hormones, or reproductive system? If you did, then ask yourself, *Am I depressed about a relationship? Frustrated about my sex life? And how about those finances—am I worried or stressed about money?*

- Or maybe you circled the third center for digestion, weight, body image, kidneys. Then you may have to sit yourself down and ask yourself, *How is that job going? What is the state of my self-esteem: do I think I'm fat? Do I hate my hair? Do I find myself attractive?*

- Or have you been having problems with sinusitis, bronchitis, lungs, heart, cholesterol, hypertension, heart palpitations, or breast lumps in the fourth center? Then you're going to have to sit yourself down and ask yourself what your partnerships are like, or your relationship to your mother or your children.

- Then we move on to the next center. Do you have neck pain, thyroid problems, TMJ problems, gum or tooth disease? Well, I hate to tell you, but communication may be an issue.

- Then there's the head, eyes, and ears. Do you have dizziness, vertigo, dry eyes, headaches, or health concerns here? You may have problems with how you see the world and your ability to change how you respond to it.

- Then there's the seventh center. We need to pause here, because these health problems will make you stop in your tracks in your life. Chronic, hard-to-treat, even life-threatening illnesses force you to focus on what your purpose in life is. Or have you lost your purpose? Have you lost your focus? And what is the quality of your spiritual life?

COMBINING MEDICAL INTUITION AND AFFIRMATIONS

So, when it comes to combining medical intuition and affirmations, we work on what I affectionately call the mind-body Bermuda Triangle. Three areas at once. We identify a scenario in our life (family, relationships, work, and so on), we identify the emotion (anger, fear, sadness, anxiety, and so on), and we identify the health problem that it involves. These are the three angles of the triangle.

However, often enough, using medical intuition and affirmations alone doesn't work. Sometimes we stay anxious or frustrated, we can't pay attention, and we still have memory problems. And a health issue may still give us trouble, despite identifying how a problem in mind or body health is associated with a scenario in our life. That's because we have to learn to support our brain and body areas physiologically, nutritionally, and possibly medicinally as they heal.

In the first book I wrote with Louise Hay—*All Is Well: Heal Your Body with Medicine, Affirmations, and Intuition,* you learned that using affirmations and intuition isn't enough. We need to use *all* solutions to heal. This book is the second in the series. It will help heal your *mind*, creating wholeness with medicine, affirmations, and intuition. It acknowledges that we need all three of these to heal.

We can combine Louise Hay's approach with medical intuition not just to tailor solutions for illnesses, but to change the thought patterns that impact our capacity to have a healthy mood, be free of anxiety and frustration, and keep our mind sharp as a tack. We can manage to have a fresh perspective on a trauma that affects our relationships and our freedom to move about the world. And when it comes to sexuality and body image and identity, we can transform our self-worth and self-esteem with affirmations as well.

HOW TO USE THIS BOOK

In *All Is Well*, Louise and I dealt with the body side of the equation—how to heal your body. This book teaches you how to heal your mind. In the chapters ahead, you will learn about your or your loved one's sadness, depression, and anger; anxiety; addiction; problems with attention and learning; healthy aging and memory; and the wide array of brain "styles" that shape the way we think and live, including unusual gifts such as mysticism.

You'll come to understand how these aspects of mental and emotional health affect your health as well. When you have a specific concern with your brain and mind, you may want to go directly to the All Is Well Clinic in the chapter about your particular problem. This is your chance to be a client in Louise's and my virtual mind-body clinic. You'll be able to determine if you have the problem by looking at a list of its symptoms in body and mind. There will be a brief example of a prototypical client's history, and then there will be a whole menu of suggestions, strategies you can employ to heal. In this way, by holding this book, you get a virtual healing experience right in your own home, with medicines, nutritional supplements, herbs, and whole-body prescriptions drawn from Louise's and my areas of expertise in helping people heal. You'll get the opportunity to bring to your healing team at home the different approaches to treatment, ranging from supplements to therapy to new behaviors, new thought patterns, and on and on.

Please understand that any solution you attempt has to be part of a healing partnership. Nurturance is part of healing, and healing cannot be done in isolation. So resist the impulse to go it alone. Take the information in this book, find a skilled, credentialed, empathic practitioner—maybe even a healer—and assemble a plan. Together, you'll use the tools in this book to help you support your brain, your mind, and your spirit so you can make the changes you want in your life.

Chapter 1

DEPRESSION

Has depression been a barrier to thriving in your life? Have sadness and frustration gotten in the way of your using all your potential at work? Have emotional pain and sensitivity disrupted your relationships?

One of the most common physical disorders in our culture is pain. One of the most common emotional disorders in our culture is emotional pain. Sadness, frustration, overwhelm: all of these have the same brain energy, or chemistry, or whatever you call it. It all comes under the heading of depression.

What is depression anyway? Depression is excessive sadness. Most people realize that. A lot of people don't realize it's also a lack of love and joy. All of us have moments of feeling abandoned, betrayed, rejected. However, if your sadness stays on for a long time, you've got an emotional problem that ends up becoming physical.

What causes the emotional pain of sadness, frustration, depression? Sometimes you feel that you've lost someone forever. Sometimes you feel worthless. Other times at work you've been disrespected. You've been treated unfairly. You'll get irritated, aggravated, thinking things should be different. This grumpiness, loneliness, and irritability are all flavors of sadness. And then your body feels it. You get hungry. You get tired. You move slowly. You find yourself slamming doors. Small things make you snap. You criticize yourself. You criticize others. And you look in the mirror and you say, "I don't like myself." You can't figure out if you're sad or if you're angry. It's difficult to know where the sadness ends, the irritability begins, and the anger erupts.

WAYS OF LOOKING AT DEPRESSION

Our feelings are an intuitive part of our well-being, letting us know that some need is not being met. When we feel sad or angry, it can overwhelm us, take over our lives, and make our relationships a battlefield. We may abuse ourselves with food, drinking, bad relationships. Often when we're in a "bad mood," we feel we're not "good enough," because depression, anger, and irritability aren't just about being in a bad mood. They're about not having enough joy and love. We can learn from Louise Hay's work that good emotional and physical health begins with loving yourself.

DEPRESSION AND MEDICAL INTUITION

In medical intuition, sadness and anger are part of your emotional guidance system, which tells you that something needs to change. Emotions themselves aren't the problem. Sadness and anger are often seen as negative. Why? Because they don't feel good. However, difficult emotions like anger and sadness are a fire alarm. Fire alarms are never pleasant. They blare in your ear, and you don't want to hear them when they go off. When you're depressed—or when you're around someone who's depressed—it's like an intuitive siren going off. Depression or sadness is an intuitive signal that something around you is about to turn out badly. When you get that overwhelming dread, that nameless discomfort inside of you, you may feel you have something to lose.

2

So the next time your mood plummets, stop. Think about it. Try to figure out why the intuitive alarm has started to go off. Is a relationship going to bite the dust? Is someone's health going to go downhill? When an emotion starts to slide into depression or irritability, intuitively we have to stop and ask ourselves what is wrong in our lives.

If you want to improve your emotional and physical health, you have to capture the intuitive message behind moods. First note the emotion, then name it, then respond to it. Let's take depression. First it appears in your right brain. That's the area for emotion and intuition. We have to take that feeling of depression and irritability from its most pure, intense form in our right brain, and transfer it to our left brain. With the left brain we can name it, find out what is causing the feeling, and decide how to respond to it effectively.

Say, for example, you're at work and all of a sudden you find you're depressed. Before you reach for that Snickers bar, or you start to snap when your co-worker hands you those files, stop yourself. Find the intuitive message behind the mood. It will prevent the depression from escalating and taking hold in your mind and body. By stopping, figuring out what you're feeling by naming it, and responding to it effectively, you're more likely to release the sadness and irritability before the mood creates a biochemical cascade. Marinating in depression creates a biochemical cascade that can result in symptoms in many areas of your body. We'll begin to describe this here, and later on in this chapter you're going to learn more about the specific chemicals of each complex emotion.

Let's look at anger, for example. What's anger? When you find yourself about to snap when someone slams the door at home, or you're frustrated when another person cuts you off on the highway, what is that feeling? It's anger. Anger is an oh-so-critical emotion. It means someone's disrespected you, or someone has threatened you. Next time you're in a line at the airport or at the grocery store or wherever you are, stop yourself. When you feel exasperated, irritated, maybe even on the verge of a full-blown rage, know that you can stop the emotion—that is, anger—in its tracks before anger's biochemistry escalates into a mind-body domino effect of health problems.

Allow yourself to sit for even a second or two with the frustration, irritation, resentment. Imagine in your mind you're switching it from the right side of your head, your right brain, to the left side of your head, your left brain. Try to find out the intuitive message behind the emotion. But better than that, try to find out what thought is keeping that anger button in your brain stuck on. Usually it's not just the line, the person cutting you off in traffic, or even the pressure of the noise and the crowds. It's usually a thought pattern like *I'm right, they're wrong, and this situation should be different.* That's true; they shouldn't cut you off in traffic. They shouldn't push you in line. The fact remains that these kinds of thoughts—the woulda, coulda, shoulda thoughts—only escalate anger in your brain and body.

Without finding the intuitive message behind the mood and transforming your thoughts, you may find yourself an hour later in a meltdown. This chapter helps you transform those moments of madness that are a part of normal life into emotional and physical health.[1]

MOOD BECOMES MEDICAL: THE EMOTIONAL DOMINO EFFECT

How does a negative emotion like sadness or anger get transformed into symptoms in your body? Mood becomes a medical problem via a domino effect of chemicals.

First: Something makes you angry, whether it's getting a bill that's too big or someone breaking up with you. Or something makes you sad. Maybe a beloved pet dies or you find out a friend is moving out of state. Whatever it is, you simply can't snap out of it. You find as the days go on that you're in a "foul mood." Or you're "down in the dumps." As the days go on, that foul mood or down-in-the-dumps feeling becomes a nameless discomfort before it becomes full-blown symptoms. Those emotions, the anger, the sadness, move down from your right brain, that area for pure emotions, to your hypothalamus.

Yes, you're right—that hypothalamus is that same area for hormones, for regulating eating and sleeping. That's why when you're in a bad mood and you stay in a bad mood for a long time, it disrupts your sleeping, your eating, and your hormones. Then the sadness and anger go to the pituitary gland. More hormonal, eating, and sleeping changes occur. And then finally, as the days and the months go by, those chemical symptoms proceed via the brain stem to your adrenal gland, which broadcasts the emotions all over your body.

Second: When you feel frustrated or depressed, your brain stem releases epinephrine, a neurotransmitter that makes you get wound up and irritable. Your adrenal gland also releases a stress hormone, cortisol, that makes you want to eat even more. Nice!

Third: That stress hormone cortisol starts those infamous immune system problems. What was first frustration and sadness now becomes a longer-term funk or depression. "Body" depression sets in with a cascade of irritating, sleep-inducing, and pain-causing cytokines. Cytokines promote inflammation everywhere in your body.

Fourth: As a result of these cytokines, your white blood cells, those immune system cells in your body, release proteins that make you feel weak, tired, and achy. You feel like you have the flu, or a fever, or arthritis.

Fifth: The cytokines "eat up" your mood neurotransmitters, making you even more depressed. Norepinephrine and serotonin, important to keep your mood elevated, start to drop, causing you to feel even more depressed, more angry, and more irritable.

Sixth: Months later, your depression and anger become more solidified in your body and organ systems, especially your heart, your blood pressure, and your blood sugar. If you went to your doctor, he or she would note that your blood homocysteine levels were beginning to rise, alerting you that you're at risk for heart disease. Your depression is now registering medical-intuitively in the form of a broken heart.

Seventh: Now changes in the neurotransmitters norepineph-rine and serotonin cause body ache, pain, everywhere. First it's in your head, then it's in your back. It's everywhere. You feel like you're dragging your body around.

Eighth: Long-term aggravation and depression start to bother you even at night. You can't fall asleep. You can't stay asleep. You can't stay awake during the day.

Ninth: Then as the months go on, as if that weren't bad enough, you start to notice that the pounds are packing on. Or you're los-ing weight, depending on your genes. If you are gaining weight, you may see that you're eating more carbohydrates—pasta, rice, sweets—and thus your weight is going up. Ultimately you might drink more alcohol to get to sleep. Both trigger a vicious cycle of more health problems.

Tenth: As your weight goes up, it causes your cholesterol to go up, increasing your risk of heart disease and stroke even more.

Eleventh: Are you still with me? Because it's getting pretty depressing. You've developed, with your weight increase, more insulin problems and more blood pressure problems. With the increased weight and increased insulin, inflammation goes up, and cholesterol floats in your blood vessels.

Twelfth: The cholesterol plus depression creates molecules called free radicals that, over time, like rust, clog up your mem-ory circuits. You notice you can't read a page of a book without reading it over and over and over again to get the meaning. You find you can't remember what you said just a few seconds ago. You can't remember people's names. Are you remembering what you just read here?

Thirteenth: Omega-3 fatty acids start to go down, and this combined with inflammation, decades later, increases your chance of dementia as well—the thought of which makes you even more depressed.

So, as you go through this book, you're going to realize that when you master finding the intuitive message behind the mood, you won't just have relief from chronic depression and irritability (this chapter) and anxiety (Chapter 2), better capacity to avoid

6

addictions (Chapter 3), better ability to learn (Chapter 4) and to remember what you've learned and age better (Chapter 5). You'll have more emotional control to fulfill all of your lifelong and spiritual potential on earth (Chapter 6).

THE SADNESS AND ANGER MIND-BODY NETWORK

Turn on the TV. All you hear about depression is medicine, medicine, medicine. You got your Prozac, you got your Lexapro, all these different medicines. Is that what depression is? Is it a Prozac deficiency? Actually, no. Depression is the sadness circuit in your brain and body gone awry.

What is the brain-body network for sadness? Let's look first at the brain. The limbic area of the brain, specifically the temporal lobe, is important for emotion and intuition. This area links our feelings and our intuition to memory in our brain and body.

We have essentially five basic emotions: anger, sadness, fear, love, and joy. In essence, depression is too much sadness and anger and too little love and joy. Medicines like Prozac, Zoloft, and Lexapro, I might add, only reduce depression, since they are antidepressants. They don't add love and joy. Affirmations, cognitive behavioral therapy, and learning how to live better teach you how to acquire love and joy.

The other part of the brain is the frontal lobe. If the limbic system is for emotions, generally speaking, the frontal lobe is for thought and action. Specifically, certain people who have had a history of trauma have memories, tapes, that their frontal lobe plays over and over when they are depressed. *I'm worthless. No one will ever love me. This is useless.* Or *I'm right, they're wrong, things should be different.* Another part of the frontal lobe helps us get up and go toward what we want when we feel joy, or gets stuck in inertia when we feel chronically depressed.

What is anger? Anger can be the first symptom of changing hormones, escalating blood pressure, not to mention an abusive relationship or past extreme trauma. We have anger management groups, but they're often court-mandated. And court-mandated therapy is rarely successful. You must know this. You can drag a horse to water, but you can't make him drink. Depression and sadness are a normal part of human experience, and so is anger. Scientists are beginning to see that the anatomy for anger and the anatomy for depression are very similar and overlapping.[2]

When you feel angry, what does it mean? That you didn't get what you wanted. You didn't get what you expected. Anger is very much associated with the temporal area but also with an area in the frontal lobe, the nucleus accumbens, the area for reward. If you don't get what you want, you get frustrated, and then it can escalate to rage, and the loop goes around and around and around. As you can see, much of the sadness network in the brain overlaps with the anger network, which is why, going back to the beginning of the chapter, we would say "I'm sad," "I'm frustrated," and then "I'm overwhelmed." Around and around. Wherever sadness and anger begin, they both end in overwhelm.

You've heard the saying that depression is anger turned inward. Maybe you saw it in some pop psychology book. Actually it isn't pop psychology; it was noted by an early psychoanalyst named Karen Horney. (That's really her last name—when I first heard it, I couldn't believe it.) Karen Horney talks about depression as anger turned inward into self-hatred. People who have that kind of depression often are born in an environment that's unpredictable and scary, where they feel helpless. In order to adapt to that frightening environment, instead of getting angry at the people around them, they get angry at themselves. It's a peculiar aspect of humanity that we do this, but we do. Instead of thinking, "My God, these people are crazy, why am I here, how could I possibly love these individuals?" they say, "I'm unlovable, I'm a bad person." To avoid getting abused, to stay out of the line of fire, they become self-effacing and submissive. They won't fight, and they become unfortunately passive. The old approach of "I'll try to get you to love me so maybe you won't hurt me" often doesn't work. Often if you're born into these kinds of abusive households, you try to earn your sense of "lovability" by feeling needed. You do everything for everyone, and then when they don't love you, you feel you're unlovable, and then you get depressed. So this is one way that depression arises from anger turned inward. Whose anger is it? Whose anger? I repeat that. Is it your anger at the people who've abused you turned inward because you couldn't express it because if you did they'd hurt you? Or do you intuitively absorb their anger by being in their environment? I'd say it is both, because now we know that depression and anger aren't just about *your* emotions but also about intuitively responding to the environment around you.

A Brief Word about Diagnosis

Much of my time in training was spent treating sadness with antidepressants as well as psychotherapy. When I started my psychiatry residency, we treated people's mood, anxiety, and other mind disorders in the following way:

1. We listened to their complaints about their mood and health.

2. We watched how they ate, slept, and acted.

3. Believe it or not, we counted symptoms, and we matched the numbers of symptoms to diagnostic categories in a manual, the guidebook to psychiatry, called the DSM-IV.

There was major depression, minor depression. Some people had bipolar I, bipolar II. The list went on. Mind you, there were no scans, X-rays, or blood tests to confirm a diagnosis as in other medical specialties, like gynecology, oncology, or internal medicine. Now, in the 21st century, guess what? We got another book with another list of different names for diagnoses. This is the DSM-V.

In the '80s, you might have had a diagnosis of ADD—attention deficit disorder. Then in the '90s someone might have thought you had Asperger's. In the early 2000s they might have said you had bipolar II. By the year 2020 or 2030, what will the diagnosis be? And what medicine will be prescribed? It's still the same brain!

Right now, most of psychiatry is based on how sad you are or how happy or anxious you are. And though we note how often patients get angry, ironically there aren't any anger diagnoses. But there are many diagnoses involving mood shifts: bipolar, borderline, and so on. Suffice it to say, this book is helping you heal your mind with every available option to date. Labels, that is, diagnoses, aren't going to be emphasized, because they're ever-changing. The brain doesn't tend to change; the labels and diagnoses sure do. They're often politicized too—we're not going to get involved with that.

DEPRESSION, ANGER, AND LOVING YOURSELF

Louise Hay looks at a solution to mood problems. She talks about how to solve the sadness and depression and anger by adding love and joy. Instead of thinking about why you don't love yourself, whether it was because someone hurt you or you were in an environment that was filled with hate, she simply tells you to love who you are. She tells you to love yourself just *where* you are. When Louise talks about loving yourself, this isn't about your waist size or your hips or your hair color. That's not love, it's vanity. And she says that is fear. Louise is talking about respecting and cherishing the incredible miracle that every single one of us is. When we love ourselves, we're loving the divine, the magnificent expressions of life. When we love ourselves, we know we are tuning in to the universe and the inherent love that flows through life. Louise sees that anger and depression and sadness are inextricably related, and many in the earlier branch of psychology called object relations agree with her.[3] This is amazing, since Louise never got a Ph.D. or did a psych residency like others have done.

Why do we have trouble loving ourselves? Let's first ask, how do we learn to love ourselves? When you're born you look up at whoever gave birth to you, you see them, they see you, and you think, *Hmm, this is love.* You absorb it in that limbic–frontal lobe network in your brain. Unfortunately if the person isn't the most loving individual, you absorb that perhaps *you* are not the most loving individual. And you end up with a little flaw in your brain. Unfortunately, that flaw may take the form of thought patterns in your frontal lobe that go around and around: *I'm not lovable. I'm not desirable. No one will love me.* So you have this little imperfection in your brain, your personality, that connects to the memory in your brain and body, and that is your self-image that ultimately ends up affecting your emotional and physical health.

Is that it for you? Is your whole life defined by that internalized image? No, it's not. There are some "theorists" who say your self-image is static. It's not true. You can change your profile. Books such as *The Confidence Code* go into exquisite detail about self-esteem and self-confidence in all their different aspects.[4] Whether it's with affirmations, cognitive behavioral therapy, or other strategies, you can always work on that corrupted file in your mind and body memory bank by altering your mood, building your sense of strength with exercise, working on spirituality, connecting to your higher power—you name it, you can change it. You can love yourself. If you want to as part of healing your mood, you can work with a therapist to help you heal the loss and grief from your early life. With the help of that therapist, that "prosthetic" mother or father, you'll be reshaping your brain and body memory banks.

DEPRESSION AND ANGER

I wish I had a dollar for everybody who called me for a medical intuitive reading who had a health problem in the depression and anger mind-body network but said they weren't depressed, angry, or unhappy. These people don't have mind depression, they have body depression. What's body depression? Instead of people experiencing sadness and anger and being able to talk about the emotion itself, they don't. They talk about it in terms of feeling tired. They feel a pressure on their chest, they can't breathe, their legs feel like lead. They can't fall asleep, they can't stay asleep. The muscles in their bodies are clamped down tight, their blood pressure is going up, their cholesterol is going up, they have an ulcer, and so on. How could this possibly be? These people are describing the symptoms they're experiencing from the neurochemical changes of that domino effect. After the cytokines have set the scene for inflammation, it's quite possible the person may experience only one-half of the domino effect of problems with depression and anger and not the other half. The neurotransmitters for depression and anger have set the scene for symptoms that are more dominant in the body than in the brain. Remember, if we can't express an emotion like sadness or anger—if we can't move it from our right brain to our left brain, name it, and respond to it—it goes down into the body as well.

Medical intuition is precisely the system that helps people with body manifestations of mind problems. When there's an emotion in our life we can't handle, our body will let us know through symptoms in specific regions. So, for example, we can look at problems in any one of the seven centers we talked about earlier:

- If you start to experience problems with your immune system, your blood, your skin, your muscles and joints, or anemia or mononucleosis, problems in the first center, you ask yourself, "What or who have I lost in a family?"

- If you have symptoms in the second center, the pelvic area, the relationship area of your body—such as PMS, vaginitis, and so on—you ask yourself, "Have I had a loss, sadness, or anger associated with a relationship or money?"

- If you have symptoms in in the third center, the midsection of your body, such as diabetes or allergies, ask yourself, "Do I have sadness about my self-esteem or work?"

- Problems in the fourth center, heart, breasts, and lungs, may have to do with grief about partnerships or children.

- In the fifth center, that hypothyroidism may come from rage about being left out.

- In the sixth center, those cataracts may be inability to see joy ahead.

- In the seventh center, that anger or hurt or long-standing resentment could be leading you to increased risk for cancer.

TREATING BODY DEPRESSION AND ANGER WITH MEDICINE

People come to me as a medical intuitive from all over the world with health problems in their brains and their bodies. Many of the nutritional supplements, herbs, and medicines that help with physical problems may also help with emotional problems. For example, many of the mood-elevating supplements or medicines like Prozac, Zoloft, or 5-HTP or SAMe may help with many immune system disorders. Why? Because they influence those immune mediators. Yes, the same immune mediators that are part of that domino effect we looked at earlier. Scientists now believe that those neuromodulators, cytokines, influence a wide range of diseases, whether it's Lyme, lupus, chronic fatigue, fibromyalgia, or rheumatoid arthritis. So whether you have depression, frustration, or any of those other disorders, the supplements and medicines to help you may be the same. If I suggest to someone that they consider rhodiola for an arthritic condition, for example, they'll say, "I know what rhodiola is for—it's for depression. You think I'm depressed and anxious." And I'll say, "No, I'm just telling you rhodiola helps with serotonin but it also helps with cortisol, and your problem is with cortisol." And usually the person then says, "Okay."[5]

THE ALL IS WELL CLINIC

The rest of this chapter is devoted to the All Is Well Clinic, where you get a virtual experience of how to heal your depression, anger, and moodiness.

I. MIND-BODY DEPRESSION AND ANGER

Chances are all of us have experienced this at one time or another in our life. But are your mind and body hanging out in a depression- and anger-filled environment right now? Look at the lists below and check off the items that seem to apply to your life now. As you do this, you're doing an intuitive reading on yourself.

MIND SYMPTOMS

- You feel grief, hurt, sorrow, loneliness, agitation, bitterness, frustration, or grouchiness.

- These feelings have become entrenched after the loss of a loved one.

- You've been disrespected by someone you care about.

- This sense of anguish may have occurred after not getting what you've worked for in a job or a career.

- You may be intuitively keyed in to someone else's depression or sadness.

- You think that life is hopeless.

- You may feel worthless.

- You blame yourself for things that go wrong around you.

- You believe you're being treated unfairly.

- You believe life should be different.

- You may want your life to end.

- You may want someone else's life to end.

BODY SYMPTOMS

- You feel tired, achy; you get repeated infections.

- You can't get your body out of bed. You sleep later and later.

- You can't get to sleep or stay asleep.

- When you move, you walk slowly and shuffle your feet.

- Your legs feel like lead and your posture is droopy.

- Your teeth clamp down and your hands are clenched.

- Your face is flushed and hot.

- You find yourself slamming doors and banging things.

- Your hormones keep going up and down; if you're a woman, your emotions are worse during the second part of your menstrual cycle or during menopause.

- If you're a man over 50, you feel exhausted and lack energy; you don't want to have sex.

- You want to eat everything, or you don't want to eat anything—you have no appetite.

- You have an empty feeling in the pit of your stomach.

- You want to drink a lot of alcohol.

- You want to spend a lot of money on things you wouldn't usually.

- You feel a lead-like pressure in your chest.

- Your blood pressure goes up and down.

- You're short of breath.

- You feel like you have a lump in your throat.

- You can't remember anything; you can't focus, or you tend to focus on one thing that makes you anxious and marinate about it.

If this is you, follow me into the All Is Well Clinic and you will see a variety of solutions that might be right for you to consider using with your healing team. Before we get to your case, though, listen to Felicia's story.

FELICIA: A SLOW DRIP OF DEPRESSION

Felicia came to the clinic because she said she felt "blah." Ironically, her name means "happiness."

THE INTUITIVE READING

I looked at Felicia. Her family was loving. No traumas, no tragedies. However, I just couldn't see any passion or purpose in Felicia's life either. It seemed like the lights were dimmed in her house. Her brain felt like she couldn't focus. She had no get-up-and-go, so I couldn't see her engaging in a career. She had no energy for hobbies, or leaving the house, or even friends. However, Felicia had people around her who were active and dramatic, and somehow this frustrated her. She seemed to feel that life was unfair because other people seemed to get happiness she couldn't attain.

THE BODY

My intuitive reading continued to Felicia's physical health. I saw that her brain lacked "battery fluid." Were there antibodies against her thyroid? She seemed sad, hopeless. Were there chronic immune system problems directed against her joints? It felt like there was a chronic drip on the back of her throat, and I could see her teeth clenched and the muscles tightened in her jaw and neck.

THE FACTS

Felicia told me she had a lifelong problem with depression and disappointment. The doctors called it dysthymia, or persistent depressive disorder. No matter what she did, she just couldn't get out of the funk. No matter what foods or supplements or medicines she tried, Felicia couldn't get "undepressed" and get rid of her grouchiness. No matter who she was with or what she did, she felt the same low energy. Felicia felt like she was dragging anchor. Why couldn't she be happy like everyone else around her?

Practitioners told Felicia she might have chronic fatigue, so she tried all those treatments. None helped. Other practitioners told her she had adrenal fatigue. Despite all the supplements she tried for cortisol, for immune system disorders, her depression was the slow drip of a faucet. Sad, sad, sad. And just a tinge of resentment. And her sadness prevented her from having normal intimacy in relationships. Some of the treatments for chronic fatigue, fibromyalgia, or adrenal fatigue worked, but eventually stopped helping. Her doctors said she had "subclinical thyroid problems," and she always felt like she had a virus.

THE SOLUTION

Do you struggle with sadness and frustration? Does happiness seem to be consistently just a little out of your reach? If you are dealing with persistent sadness and low energy, that funk will eventually increase your chance toward a variety of health problems such as immune system disorders, pain, and estrogen, adrenal, and thyroid imbalances, to name just a few. If you treat just the body, like Felicia, and not the mood, health is not achieved. If you treat just the mood, the depression and irritability, you still suffer from symptoms in your body. Why? To treat brain-body depression and anger, you have to treat your whole being. Sadness and anger occur simultaneously in the brain and body. These emotions are like a brush fire. If sustained, they create inflammation in your immune system. The brain-body inflammation of depression and anger causes heat, pain, and redness that can make your joints ache. You might have problems with focus, attention, and brain fog too.

How do we know there is such a thing as a brain-body mood disorder? Depression occurs in so many inflammatory diseases. Many of the markers of body inflammation also occur in depression. So we don't just look at supporting your brain, we also support your body. Using supplements, medicines, and affirmations to address sadness, frustration, and inflammation in the brain and body can help give you the capacity to engage more fully, to enjoy more exuberance in life. And by treating your mood, we don't just give you greater emotional health, we also treat the inflammation in your body. In fact, many antidepressants have been known to lower inflammation in the body and improve the immune system.

What about therapy? Where does therapy fit into this? People with dysthymia or that long, slow burn of depression, irritability, and anger are best helped with cognitive behavioral therapy. What is cognitive behavioral therapy? Just that. Looking at the thoughts—cognitive—and identifying how they affect behavior. With a trusted counselor in cognitive behavioral therapy, we learn to name those thought patterns that are "downers," that lower our mood, and we also identify those actions that equally dampen our depression. Does this sound like affirmations? Well, yes, you're right. Many affirmations in Louise Hay's work identify a negative thought pattern and replace the depressive idea with a more positive, loving, joyful, affirming one.

THE MEDICINES

In addition, for many people, we need to also support the mood with nutritional supplements, herbs, or in some cases, if life-saving, medicine. Only you can decide with your practitioner what is right for you. This is not something to be done alone. When you have a baby, you do it in partnership. When you want to rebirth your brain and body, it's also better to do it in partnership. So, with a caring professional, look at what nutritional supplements, herbs, even hormones and medicines may be right for you to reconstitute your brain chemistry.

Right now, no one really knows what medicines and supplements are really beneficial for this form of dysthymia or persistent depressive disorder. However, there is an intense interaction between you, the patient, and the caregiver who is treating you. So don't isolate. Get help. The interaction between you and your caregiver releases opiates, a mood-elevating neurotransmitter that in itself can improve your mood. That molecule of caring, "the placebo effect," isn't just in your head. It's in your body. Those opiates that form the "glue" of empathy between people also affect immune system inflammation in your body. So get up, make that phone call. Get that first connection of help for healing.

If your depression is paralyzing, maybe even life-threatening, don't say an automatic no to medicine. Yes, you may think medicines aren't the right thing for you. Maybe you want to take a more "natural" approach. But before you write medication off completely, stop. Think. In diabetes, for many people, the pancreas stops making insulin, an important hormone—or if you prefer, neurotransmitter—that is important for brain and body chemistry. Similarly, our brain stems make neurotransmitters for our moods, and in some individuals, their brain stems for whatever reason stop making these neurotransmitters. You wouldn't think it was un-spiritual for a diabetic to take his or her insulin, would you? It's important to understand that we all need to make a choice, and for some, medicine may be that choice, whether in the short term or the long term.

So when it comes to medicine, what are the choices? They include Prozac, Zoloft, Paxil, Lexapro, and other antidepressants called tricyclic antidepressants. On the other hand, there are all these newer antidepressants that hit those other neurotransmitters that I talked about in the brain stem. Serotonin and norepinephrine are affected by Effexor, Cymbalta, and others. Many of these medicines also act on body depression, body inflammation. For one, Cymbalta affects the inflammation in the joints of people with chronic fatigue. On the other hand, there are newer medicines that you're going to hear about, such as Abilify and others, that affect both the dopamine and serotonin areas. They are important for unusual combinations of anxiety and depression. Finally, there are these seldom used but extremely effective medicines called MAO inhibitors (monoamine oxidase inhibitors, such as Nardil or Parnate). These can be very good for treating long-term depression, but they require a special diet.

But maybe you're not ready for medicines. You need to let your doctor know that, or your physician, or your practitioner, or your nurse practitioner, whoever you want to go see. You have choices:

- Consider SAMe, 400 milligrams a day on an empty stomach, or 5-HTP or rhodiola, 100 milligrams one to four times a day, but you have to make sure you don't have bipolar disorder before taking these. Ask your practitioner.

- Multivitamins: B6 and B12 are critical for serotonin production. L-methylfolate 15 milligrams for 60 days also helps people with depression.[6]

- Genetic testing: There's a movement lately toward genetic testing to determine what medication or nutritional supplement may be best for you. Whether it's determining your P450 enzyme profile, your MAO(A) subtype, and so on, people are running to "get their genes tested," especially if initial treatments haven't healed their mood problems. Yes, our health may in part be determined by genes, but there are far more "epigenetic" influences, life experiences, that may determine whether our genes even matter. In medicine, we learn to treat people, not "numbers." So resist the impulse to believe that getting long panels of blood tests is going to find your answer. Statistically, the more tests they run, the more likely this shotgun approach will yield a false positive, detecting something wrong whether it's relevant or not.

Brain fog? Problems focusing? Many supplements that work for mood also work for these symptoms:

- Ginkgo biloba 240 milligrams helps focus and attention. Beware—ask your practitioner whether it's safe due to its blood-thinning effect.

- Siberian ginseng: for balancing cortisol, adrenal, and other types of fatigue as well as focus and attention.

- Chocolate contains phenylethylalanine (PEA); it boosts motivation and energy, because it increases dopamine.

Other Treatments for Depression

Long-term changes in neurotransmitters that affect mood can affect the immune system in the body as well. Acupuncture and Chinese herbs can help that body inflammation. So if you, like Felicia, have body depression—whether it's chronic fatigue, pain, or other symptoms—go to an acupuncturist or a Chinese herbalist and look into having treatment for your spleen, stomach, and kidney meridian. You can also ask your acupuncturist for herbs, such as os draconis, that help relieve depression and body aches as well as insomnia.

Although your depression could be causing you immense fatigue, try working with a trainer or coach to rehabilitate your adrenal gland so you can have more aerobic fitness. For the first week, you may be able to exercise only 5 minutes a day, then the next week, 10 minutes a day, and so on, working your way up to 20 to 30 minutes each day. By doing this, you are also releasing opiates, which elevate your mood and your immune system.

Watch TV or movies that help you laugh, laugh, laugh! On the other hand, don't watch TV or movies that make you cry, cry, cry! It's obvious. And hang out with people who make you laugh, laugh, laugh! Don't always hang out with people who are down. Why? We know that one of the causes of depression is hanging out with depressing people. I'm not saying you kick your friends to the curb if they're having a down moment; I'm just saying, do a thorough inventory of your life. Ask your counselor if there are any chronic black holes in relationships in your life that need to be excavated.

Speaking of black holes, get out of the house! Make sure you have contact with at least one person each day, and we're not talking about the mailman here. Go to a coffee place or recreational center or spiritual center—any place where there are people you can just talk with, hang out with. Isolation is a friend of depression. Don't isolate—relate!

Get a massage. It releases neurotransmitters that improve your mood and immune system.

Connect with your spirituality, whether it's by working with a spiritual adviser, walking in nature, praying, meditating, or even just sitting in a meditative stance. Any way you contact the divine makes you feel whole and lets you know it's going to all be okay.

Ask your practitioner if you have a "seasonal" problem with your mood. What's a seasonal problem? It means that during a certain time of the year, fall or winter, your mood plummets. If this is happening to you, get a full-spectrum light source, which is easy to find in almost any health food store.

THE AFFIRMATIONS

Love is the opposite of depression, so Louise encourages people who are depressed to learn how to love themselves. Try following these ten steps she lays out:

1. Stop all criticism. Stop criticizing yourself now and forever more. Never again! Criticism never changes a thing, so refuse to criticize yourself and accept yourself exactly as you are.

2. Don't scare yourself, please. If you love yourself, don't scare yourself. Stop terrorizing yourself with frightful thoughts, because all you do is make your situation worse. Don't take a small situation and make it a big monster.

3. Be gentle and kind and patient with yourself. Just be gentle, kind, and patient. You know, a good example of the power of patience is a garden. A garden begins with just a patch of dirt. Then you add small seeds or some little plants, and you water it, and you give it some loving attention. And to begin with, it seems like not much is happening. But if you continue doing that, and if you're patient, things will change. The garden will grow and blossom. If you think of your life or your mind as like a garden, you know what kind of garden you

would like. What kind of events do you want to happen in your life, and what kinds of seeds do you need to plant in order for those to happen? Select the seeds, the thoughts, that will grow the garden of experiences you want.

4. Be kind to your mind. You know, self-hatred is really only hating thoughts you have about yourself. And you don't want to hate yourself for having thoughts. You gently want to change those thoughts. You are worth loving. All of us are.

5. Praise yourself. Please praise yourself. Criticism breaks down the inner spirit and praise builds it up. So praise yourself as much as you can. Tell yourself how well you're doing with every little thing. Many of us refuse to put any effort into creating a good life for ourselves, because we feel we don't deserve it. Our feeling of not being deserving could be from people telling us we aren't, but it could also be from something as simple as early toilet training or being refused an ice-cream cone when we were young. Deserving has nothing to do with having good. It's our willingness to accept good in our lives. Allow yourself to accept good whether you think you deserve it or not.

6. Find ways to support yourself. Reach out to friends and allow them to help you. It really is being strong to ask for help when you need it, instead of trying to do it all yourself and then being angry at yourself because you can't make it. And there are so many ways. Friends can help you. There are support groups everywhere, and if you can't find what you want, you can even start your own.

7. Be loving to your negatives. You created every single negative pattern, every negative habit. Everything you have in your life, you created to fulfill a need,

and it worked. See, everybody has made negative choices in the past. However, nobody is stuck with them. The good news is that you always have a choice. You can always choose to let go of the old pattern, and you can choose a different, more supportive and nourishing thought. Letting go of the old negative pattern with love allows you to move into the new positive patterns with ease.

8. Take care of your body. It's the house you live in. When you're born, you move into this house, and when you leave the planet, you move out of it. So, love the house that you live in and take care of it. You can find exercise that you enjoy, something that's fun to do, and then watch what you put in your body. Drug abuse is so prevalent on the planet, it's become one of the most popular methods of escape. If you're into drugs, it doesn't mean you are a bad person. It just means that you haven't found a more positive way of fulfilling your needs. But drugs alter our reality and lower our immune system to dangerous levels. Instead of escaping with drugs, we need to know that it is safe for us to feel our feelings. Part of loving ourselves is feeling our feelings. And they pass through, they don't stay.

9. Do mirror work. I have seen so many people change their lives by merely looking in the mirror and saying, "I love you. I really love you." At first it may seem untrue or weird, and it can bring up sadness or anger or fear, but if you continue to do this simple affirmation every time you're in front of a mirror, your inner energy begins to shift. You're letting go of destructive thoughts and behaviors, and accepting yourself as naturally lovable becomes so much easier.

10. There are several ways you can practice mirror work. First thing in the morning, I like just looking in the

mirror and saying, "I love you. What can I do for you today to make you happy?" Then listen to what you hear. You may not get any messages to begin with, because you may be so used to beating yourself up that you don't know how to respond to a kind, loving thought, but listen and follow through and begin to learn to trust yourself. And if something unpleasant happens, run immediately to the mirror and say, "I love you! I love you anyway!" Because events come and go, but the love that you have for yourself is constant and is the most important thing in your life.

11. You can do forgiveness work in the mirror. Look in your own eyes and say, "I forgive you. I forgive you for holding on to old patterns for too long. I forgive you for not loving yourself. I forgive you for whatever." You can talk to other people in the mirror too. Tell people in the mirror what you are afraid to say in person. You can forgive them. You can ask for love and approval. It's a wonderful way to talk to your parents or your partner in a relationship. Talk to your doctor in the mirror. Talk to your boss in the mirror. You can say all kinds of things you would be afraid to say otherwise. Be sure the last thing you say in the mirror is always that you love and approve of yourself.

12. The most important thing is to just be willing. Just be willing. Say, "I am willing to learn to love myself. I'm willing to learn to love myself. I'm willing." And believe me, the universe will hear you.

II. Roller-Coaster Moods

Cycles of mood can include all the symptoms of depression and anger that we saw in the previous section. What we add here is now-you-see-it-now-you-don't moods. And we also have now-you-see-it-now-you-don't health problems that are inextricably related to mood, seemingly unrelated to life experience. In addition to roller-coaster moods, you have roller-coaster symptoms in your body, ups and downs of health and disease seemingly unrelated to your health practices. You seem to be sailing along, relatively happy, and then the bottom falls out. Not only do you become depressed and frustrated (who wouldn't?), you're also sick in multiple areas of your body. And then for a variety of reasons you get relief, only to repeat the cycle a month or two later. Often enough the cycles of happiness get shorter and shorter and the unpleasant cycles get longer and longer.

Some people would call your roller-coaster moods "bipolar-esque," that is, swings from sadness to joy to irritability to anger, around and around. That is, your brain has some problem maintaining your mood on an even keep without wild swings from depression to excessive joy—mania—to rage, irritability, or the so-called mixed states. I think there's also such a thing as bipolar body disorder—that the neurochemistry in your body can have a similar problem with balance. Seemingly unprovoked by what you eat, what supplements, treatments, or medicines you take, your body has a problem maintaining that status-quo balance of day-to-day health, and of course this makes sense. Many of the neurochemicals that influence immune system hormones, digestion, allergy, the cardiovascular system, and so on are the same neurochemicals that influence depression, sadness, joy, anger, love, and fear. So if your brain has problems with the mechanism that maintains balance, your body probably has the same balance problem as well.

Look at the following lists of symptoms, in addition to the lists from the previous section, and check off the ones that apply to your life right now.

MIND SYMPTOMS

- Your usual good mood slumps for no good reason into hurt, rejection, and gloom.

- Your normal mood, for no reason, becomes just a little too cheerful, exhilarated, and optimistic in a way that doesn't seem to match what's going on in your current circumstances. Your mood doesn't match the circumstances.

- In contrast to your normal even-keeled mood, you begin to talk over people, not sleep, and feel driven to busy yourself with shopping, buying, working, driving fast, and even engaging in risky sexual relationships and business investments.

- Your thoughts go rapid-fire and you start to act on impulse, the opposite of your usual common sense.

- You fly off the handle for seemingly no reason whatsoever. Your irritability and moodiness escalate to the point where you find yourself having more and more arguments with people in a way you wouldn't ordinarily.

BODY SYMPTOMS

- You have ups and downs in your health that don't seem to be related to your health practices.

- You're sick in multiple areas of your body, perhaps experiencing infections, allergies, pain, digestive issues, or problems with hormonal imbalance.

- Your body has difficulty maintaining balance day to day, in ways that seem unrelated to what you eat or what supplements or medicines you take.

Is this you? Have you been chasing roller-coaster changes in your body of infections, allergies, pain, digestive problems, or estrogen, testosterone, or thyroid hormone levels, to name a few? If the ups and downs of these health problems along with simultaneous cycles of depression, frustration, elation, and so on, are getting you down, read on.

GALENA: CYCLES OF MOOD

Galena called me for a reading. She told me that a friend had suggested she needed it.

THE INTUITIVE READING

Galena's life seemed like it contained a fogged-up mirror, a distorted image of herself. Why? When she was about seven or eight, somehow her self-image had been bruised. Was it that someone said she was fat? Or ugly? I didn't know. I had a hard time seeing relationships. When I looked at Galena's family, I could see her always taking care of everyone. Was that how she felt that she was lovable?

THE BODY

When I looked intuitively at Galena's body, her digestive tract seemed to go up and down like a balloon inflating and deflating. Galena's moods seemed to go up and down as well. Irritability and moodiness changed to anxiety and being keyed up. Galena's body appeared to have that "red tinge" of estrogen excess/deficient progesterone. I sensed increased body fat stores and problems with insulin. I saw problems with irregular periods and tiny cysts in her ovarian area. Galena's periods seemed to alternate between being very heavy and being completely absent. I saw frequent breakouts in her skin. Whether it was her digestion, her weight, or her skin, Galena's health seemed to be intertwined with moods that would plummet when people rejected her. Her moods seemed to be as reactive as her hormones.

THE FACTS

Galena told me she had had PMS since she was in puberty, and now at 48, she suffered from what they call perimenopause. She laughed and said she had been "perimenopausal for 20 years." She complained that her family said her moods "cycled with the moon." Her happiness waxed and waned along with her hormones. Doctors said that her 30 to 40 pounds of excess weight caused her to have polycystic ovary disease, and that was the cause of her moodiness and irritability. Whether it was the acne or the weight, Galena was really concerned about her body image and how it affected her relationships. Galena wanted to know what to do with her lifelong problem with mood swings and hormones.

The Solution

Are you, like Galena, concerned about roller-coaster moods and continual ups and downs in your health? Women are twice as likely as men to have depression and twice as likely to have cyclic health problems like lupus, hypothyroidism, and irritable bowel syndrome (IBS). And women are more likely to have seasonal patterns of mood, not to mention more rapid cycling of mood swings. Is that due to hormonal ups and downs? No one knows. All we do know is there's an incredible interconnection between ups and downs in neurotransmitters that affect mood and ups and downs in health problems you may be struggling with. In our culture now, enough people are being diagnosed with bipolar disorder or bipolar II (that is, unstable moods) that, given the intricate connections and chemistry between brain and body, it's only a matter of time before we realize there are bipolar body problems as well.

If you are concerned with unstable moods as well as unstable hormones and other health problems, the first step is to stabilize brain and body. You may have noted that some of your mood problems, specifically mood swings, "run in your family," and maybe genetically you are predisposed to a lot of the health problems you have as well. Maybe the women or men in your family were prone to hormonal and reproductive problems, thyroid disorders, and cyclic changes in IBS, digestive allergies, and so on. We are not at the mercy of our genes, though, whether for brain or body problems. There are problems that occur in our families, work, and relationships that can switch on our depression just like there are switches in our genes that can switch off depression. And we can train our brain with cognitive behavioral therapy, nutritional supplements and medicine, changes in diet, and regulating body fat to learn how to switch off the mood and health-problem genes.[7]

For example, how does mood affect fat content? How does that work? Your adrenal gland takes the body fat and converts it via progesterone to excess estrogen. Too much estrogen is depressing. We know this because when you take an oral contraceptive pill, one of the side effects is depression. On the other hand, excessive body fat can cause "body depression," because it causes inflammation. If you have excessive body fat (more than 40 pounds), you may have an increased chance toward both—estrogen dominance and body inflammation, not to mention depression. And excess body fat raises insulin, increases your chance toward polycystic ovary disease, and disrupts your menstrual cycle. Up and down we go on the roller coaster.

STABILIZING BRAIN–BODY HORMONES

I recommend you see a complementary nutritionist who can help you create an eating plan to regulate your blood sugar. You can also try this five-meal-a-day eating plan yourself:

- Breakfast: Have the equivalent of two eggs, a half slice of bread (gluten-free if you want), a bottle of water, and then exercise on an elliptical trainer or exercise bicycle for half an hour.

- 10 A.M.: Have half of a protein bar and another bottle of water.

- 12 noon: The biggest meal of the day. Take a plate and divide into thirds—one-third protein, one-third carbs, one-third vegetable. If you want dessert, which I highly suggest, take some of the carbohydrate away and have half a piece of dessert.

- 3 P.M.: Have the other half of that protein bar and your third and final bottle of water.

- Dinner: Smallest meal of the day. Small piece of protein, dark leafy vegetable. If you can walk after dinner, you'll lose the weight.

These changes in blood sugar will ultimately affect cortisol, body fat, thyroid hormone, estrogen, and other hormones in your body.

While you're on a food plan, put yourself on a responsibility diet as well. Excessive food, excessive calories make you gain weight. Carrying excessive responsibility via cortisol does the same. For every hour you do things for your family, devote an hour to doting on yourself. Beware: this will make you extremely anxious. Get a coach to help you do this. What do I mean by doting on yourself? Hair, nails, hobbies, TV, exercise, whatever brings you joy. You may feel anxious. You may feel very guilty. But you will love it when you start to lose weight.

SUPPLEMENTS AND MEDICINES

There's a range of supplements and medicines that can buffer the highs and lows of moods and hormones in your brain and body. Before you take any supplements, like rhodiola, Siberian ginseng, SAMe, or Wellbutrin, or use any stimulant, even a full-spectrum light, ask your doctor. If you have true mania, it could swing your mood into dangerous levels of up and down. Otherwise, try:

- Rhodiola 100 milligrams three or four times a day.

- Siberian ginseng 300 to 625 milligrams a day.

- SAMe 400 milligrams two or three times a day can give you energy, suppress your appetite, and help you lose weight.

- Calcium and magnesium can help to stabilize mood.

- Is hormone replacement your answer to PMS and midlife moodiness, physical symptoms, and weight problems? If you are 40 or more pounds overweight, your body fat stores provide you with excessive amounts of estrogen, so you may want to think twice about taking bioidentical estrogen or progesterone. Bioidentical progesterone, although helping stabilize your mood, in some cases may be converted to estrogen in your body and increase your chance toward a variety of dangerous health problems. You already have too much estrogen stored in your body fat, and although a physician may test your saliva or blood for estrogen and find it to be low, that's not where estrogen is stored.

- Consider a check of your thyroid hormone. People with moodiness are notorious for having thyroid disorders. T3, a form of thyroid hormone, also can be added to enhance the effect of mood stabilization treatment.

- Evening primrose oil can help with PMS and perimenopausal irritability. However, don't take it if you have a family history of breast cancer.

- DHA 1,000 milligrams three times a day can help with moodiness, not to mention a variety of immune, digestive, and other up-and-down health problems.

- Many weight-loss physicians use combinations of Wellbutrin (an antidepressant) and Topamax (a mood stabilizer) to help people lose weight. If you are moody and depressed and have tried everything else, talk to your physician.

- If you're already on an antidepressant, talk to your practitioner about whether or not, as a side effect, that medicine may make you *gain* weight. Many of them do.

- Other antidepressants that may be prescribed to help with depression include Abilify, Viibryd, Zyprexa, Latuda, Saphris, and others. By the time this book is on the shelves, there will probably be three or four new ones. All these medicines help buffer dopamine, serotonin, and norepinephrine.

- If you really have profound mind-body swings of mood and health problems, talk to a doctor

about other possible mood stabilizers: Lamictal,
Neurontin, Tegretol, and others can balance mood
and also help with ups and downs of pain and other
physical symptoms.

Go to an acupuncturist and Chinese herbalist to help balance
your liver meridian, that area of your energy system that smooths
mood and hormonal levels. Herbs like cinnabar may help with
moodiness, irritability, and skin problems.

While we're talking about herbs in general, consider chaste-
berry, vitex agnus-castus, and other herbs that can help with perimenopausal, menopausal, or PMS moodiness and irritability. These
herbs help reduce excess estrogen. They elevate progesterone and
ultimately ease hormonal moodiness, breast tenderness, and fluid
retention. The added benefit is that these mood-balancing hormones help with constipation, headache, and fatigue.

How do they work?

- Vitex helps with the neurotransmitter dopamine.

- Black cohosh helps with hot flashes by having an
  estrogen effect.

- Licorice, another herb, may help with depression's
  effect on attention.

- Dong quai, or *Angelica sinensis*, is not just good for
  menopausal symptoms but can also help with the
  melancholy and sadness.

- Finally, red clover, or *Trifolium pratense*, also has a
  mild antidepressant effect but can help improve
  osteoporosis.

THE AFFIRMATIONS

Louise suggests the following affirmations to help lift mood
and energy:

- When you feel like a failure, say this affirmation in
  the mirror: "My life is a success."

- When you want to hide under the covers, the affirmation is "I now go beyond my old fears and limitations."

- When loneliness is particularly intense, the affirmation is "I am safe. It's only change."

- When you feel anger that you feel you don't have the right to have, the affirmation is "I now go beyond other people's fears and limitations. I create my own life."

- When your energy is low, the affirmation is "I am filled with energy and enthusiasm. My body heals rapidly. I give myself permission to be well."

- When the negative thought pattern in premenstrual syndrome is allowing confusion to reign, giving power to outside influences, the affirmation is "I now take charge of my mind and life. I am a powerful, dynamic woman. Every part of my body functions perfectly. I love me."

- For menstrual problems in general, which may stem from difficult feelings about being a woman, the affirmation is "I accept my power as a woman, and accept all my bodily processes as normal and natural. I love and approve of myself."

III. TRAUMA AND MIND–BODY MOOD PROBLEMS

Have you been predisposed to depression, irritability, or moodiness due to severe trauma? In addition to the symptoms we outlined in the previous two sections, look at the lists below and check off the items that apply to your life right now.

MIND SYMPTOMS

- You experienced painful emotional or physical trauma in your family growing up.

- You've suffered emotional or physical trauma in one or more of your relationships.

- There has been an event in your life in which you've been threatened with such serious physical or emotional harm that it would be out of the range of what we consider normal life experience. Some examples might be living through war, witnessing an accident with loss of life or limb, experiencing rape or incest, or seeing your children suffer abuse.

- Whatever the trauma you've experienced, you tend to have "repeat performances" of this painful pattern in one relationship after another, one job after another, and so on. The painful pattern seems to replay over and over in your life like the movie *Groundhog Day*.

BODY SYMPTOMS

- You're exhausted all the time.

- You're jumpy, with an exaggerated startle response.

- You're hypervigilant, always scanning your environment for fear the trauma will recur.

- Many of the muscles in your body are tight like rubber bands.

- You have trouble falling asleep or staying asleep.

- You've been accident-prone since childhood.

- You've had one health problem after another since childhood.

- You tend to get autoimmune illnesses.

- You take chances and tend to be reckless or self-destructive.

- You say "I'm sorry" a lot, or you say to yourself *I am bad*, or *No one can be trusted*, or *The world is dangerous*.

- You blame yourself a lot for things that happen around you.

- You have swings of emotion; you're emotionally reactive to even the slightest changes in your environment. Whether it's anger, irritation, guilt, shame, despondency, or elation, your moods cycle rapidly depending on what's going on around you.

- You tend to feel detached from others because at times this feels safer.

- You have problems with concentration and memory.

- When things around you are intensely painful, it's easy for you to feel detached or "leave your body."

Does this list of mind-body symptoms tend to occur with you? Then perhaps a series of life experiences has altered your mind-body pathways for mood. Consider the following intuitive reading.

HETTY: MY RELATIONSHIPS ARE FALLING APART AND SO AM I

Hetty came to me because she was having a hard time managing her emotions, her health, and her relationships.

THE INTUITIVE READING

Hetty's mind seemed to be like a bundle of emotions. Fear turned into anger turned into sadness turned into joy, then love. I couldn't figure out where one emotion ended and the next one began. Whether it was fear, anger, sadness, or even love or joy, it was hard for her to name the emotion she was experiencing, respond to it effectively, and release it. When I looked at her life, I could see a kaleidoscope of relationships from childhood to adulthood, each seemingly a replay of a similar theme—that is, hurt, then escape.

The Body

Feelings seemed to pass down into Hetty's body like a waterfall. Whether it was pressure in her chest, irregular digestion, fatigue, or spurts of energy, Hetty's brain and body felt like one of those sprinklers in the front yard—first it was on, then it was off, on, off, an irregular flow.

The Facts

Hetty told me she had been diagnosed with bipolar II and post-traumatic stress disorder (PTSD). She had a history of abuse in childhood, then later on a string of relationships with partners who would emotionally and physically abuse her. Ever since she could remember, her moods would go up, then down. Her body would be physically energized, and then she would be sleeping and exhausted for days.

Trauma and Mind-Body Moodiness

How do over-the-top painful events disrupt mood and health? The horror of trauma releases cortisol, which makes your mood go up and down. Precipitous emotional and physical injury makes your brain and body release epinephrine, which initially energizes you, then makes you irritable and exhausted. The epinephrine makes the muscles in your body into tight rubber bands; you're jittery, hypervigilant, impulsive, and maybe even a little manic. The cortisol causes you to have brain fog, problems with focus and attention. And over time, trauma changes the memory pathways in your brain (more on that later) to, believe it or not, encourage you to be attracted to scenarios that repeat the traumatic event. These "do-overs" are your brain-body's way of trying to heal the past, but they only drive trauma deeper into your brain and body, making your health veer even farther off course.

If you're moody, as in the previous case we looked at, you may in psychiatry be given a diagnosis of bipolar I or bipolar II, or that nebulous condition called borderline personality disorder. Physicians and scientists now know that many people who suffer moodiness also have a history of trauma. So if you have both a history of serious emotional and physical abuse *and* mood swings, it's best to treat both problems rather than focus on a diagnostic label.

THE SOLUTION

We talked a lot about how to handle moodiness in the previous cases, so you can return there to read about those solutions.

In addition, if you have problems with moodiness and irritability, medicines and supplements aren't your only solution for the roller-coaster moods. You can learn how to rewire the two brain areas for buffering emotion: the limbic or temporal lobe area for pure emotion and the frontal lobe executive area for curbing emotion. Two treatments that help rewire these two brain regions are cognitive behavioral therapy (CBT) or dialectical behavioral therapy (DBT). Dialectical behavioral therapy, pioneered by a woman named Marsha Linehan, based on Tibetan Buddhism and mindfulness, helps you take right brain emotions and intuition and balance them with left brain thoughts to attain more balanced emotional states. DBT has been used for mood problems like bipolar, depression, anxiety, and PTSD, not to mention all those vague personality disorders that are so controversial and hard to diagnose definitively (e.g., borderline personality disorder).

Depending on the emotions you're mostly concerned about, you can tailor this work specifically for you. CBT or DBT can help you learn how to handle your anger so it doesn't cause moods to escalate. These treatments can also teach you how to effectively speak your mind to a loved one in a timely fashion and not hold in your emotions to the point where you explode into rage. You can learn how to choose an appropriate volume—not too loud, not too submissive, but something in between—and choose your words with social savvy and smoothness to say the right thing to the right person at the right time in the right way. You might ask, "How can anyone possibly learn how to do this?" I assure you, I've taken DBT and I've taught it, and I *am* learning how to do this. So can you.

Along with DBT, you can balance your mood and health with yoga and other movement practices, since they help balance initiative and motivation and help alleviate mild depression.

THE AFFIRMATIONS

Louise offers some wonderful tools for alleviating anger and building positive feelings. One is a thankful list:

> Spend 10 minutes every morning being thankful for all the good in your life. What are you grateful for? How do you begin each day? What is the first thing you say in the morning? List at least 10 things in your life that you are grateful for. Close your eyes and really think before you write. It may take you a month to write this. That's okay. There is no time limit, and you can add to the list at any time. The point is that it's hard to be grateful and angry at the same time.

Or try this exercise to create positive feelings:

> Write 50 positive feelings about yourself. It's hard to write positive feelings about yourself when you're angry, but this helps neutralize the anger. Pay attention to your feelings while you're doing the exercise. Is there resistance? Is it hard to see yourself in a positive light? Continue on, remembering how powerful you are.

And consider the following affirmations for different forms that anger may take:

- For times when you feel that anger is bad: "Anger is normal and natural."

- When someone is angry and you get scared: "I comfort my inner child. We are safe."

- When you feel it's not safe to be angry: "I am safe. It is only an emotion."

- When the thought is your parents won't allow you to express your anger: "I move beyond my parents' limitations."

- When the thought is you won't be loved if you get angry: "The more honest I am, the more I am loved."

- If you think you have to hide your anger: "I express my anger in appropriate ways."

- If stuffing anger is making you sick: "I allow myself the freedom of my emotions."

- If you think your anger is out of control: "I am at peace with myself and life."

- If you think everyone is against you: "I am lovable and everyone loves me."

- If you are afraid of anger: "I acknowledge all my feelings. It is safe for me to recognize my anger."

- If you think you have no right to be angry: "All of my emotions are acceptable."

- If you are one of those rare people who think, *I have never been angry*: "Healthy expression of anger keeps me healthy."

- If you think if you get angry, you will hurt someone: "Everyone is safe with me when I express my emotion."

- And finally: "I give myself permission to acknowledge my emotions."

IV. MOOD DISORDERS AND BRAIN FOG

Has your mind been taken hostage by depression and fog? Depression can occur alongside a "fog" that spreads from brain to body. What are the signs? Look at this list of symptoms and see which apply to your life right now.

MIND SYMPTOMS

- You find yourself precipitously sad, irritable, or annoyed for seemingly no reason whatsoever.

- You tend to lose focus and attention and get disoriented. You might be driving and realize you don't know why you're on that particular street.

- You lose clarity and speed in your thinking; your memory seems like it's clouded.

- Your friends say you talk more than usual but don't get to the point as much.

Body Symptoms

- Your arms and legs feel shaky or tremulous.

- You're sleepy during the day and up at night.

- You see things out of the corner of your eye, like moving shadows.

- You feel restless, needing to pace or move around for no reason.

- Your symptoms are unstable, meaning they can change from hour to hour and day to day; they tend to get worse around 4 P.M.

If you have a number of these symptoms, you may have brain fog. People have called it by a variety of names—confusion, delirium, befuddlement—but most people just know the phrase *brain fog*. Continue to the following case and see if it rings a bell.

Irene: I Want My Brain Back

Irene came to me for a medical intuitive reading saying, "I want my brain back."

The Intuitive Reading

When I looked at Irene's mind intuitively, I saw her thoughts come to a halt. Like a car that has stalled after stopping at a stoplight, her thoughts had simply gotten stuck. It seemed like her life had stopped as well. I couldn't see a job, couldn't see a relationship, and had trouble seeing her leave home, actually. I had trouble seeing a companion. I had trouble seeing friends, colleagues. It felt like Irene was exiled.

THE BODY

Irene seemed to have problems with forgetfulness, focus, and attention. Intuitively, she seemed to experience dizziness and a problem with disorientation when she tried to read or watch TV over time. Her whole body seemed to ache, especially her neck. She seemed sad, but she seemed to actually minimize her physical problems. Intuitively, I sensed numbness and tingling on the left side of her body, especially her hands and feet, which felt like they were asleep.

THE FACTS

Irene had been diagnosed with multiple sclerosis, but she said the doctors were full of baloney. She said, "I want my brain back." Recently she said she had fallen on the pavement, and the doctor did an MRI and found all kinds of plaques in her brain. Because of the fall and mistakes at work, she'd been forced into early retirement. Irene, an accountant, always took pride in being perfect in her work. She just couldn't understand why people were finding mistakes. Recently, Irene had been staying home and offering to take care of her grandchildren. However, her family was calling less and less due to some confusion over "mistakes" she'd made during a recent babysitting stint.

THE SOLUTION

You needn't have a serious illness to have brain fog. There are a number of areas in your mind and body where problems can cause depression, confusion, and delirium:

- Infection; immune system problems like Lyme, flu, pneumonia, or viruses; autoimmune problems like rheumatoid arthritis, lupus, and so on; cancers and tumors

- Hormonal changes in menopause or perimenopause; changes in thyroid hormone, cortisol, or testosterone, to name a few

- Unstable blood sugar

- Medicines, medicines, medicines! Be they pain pills, sleeping pills, steroids, or antidepressants, so many medicines can cause brain fog as a side effect. A variety of herbs may do the same; just because it's natural doesn't mean it can't cause brain fog. Combinations of medicines can cause brain fog as well. So can other drugs—alcohol, cocaine, marijuana, any type of drug that alters your mind.

- Changes in your body chemistry—sodium, potassium, calcium, and so on

- Eating disorders; anorexia

- Sleep apnea; unstable asthma

- Cardiovascular disease; after a heart attack or heart surgery; unstable hypertension; blood pressure medications

- Seizure disorders; brain problems like Alzheimer's disease and other dementia; brain injury, concussions, bleeds; other brain disorders, such as multiple sclerosis

- Surgery, anesthesia, or combinations of serious illnesses

- Emotional trauma

- Spiritual illumination and ecstatic states

So the solution to your brain fog will obviously depend on the cause of your brain fog.

What is the treatment for brain fog and mood disorders? You treat the physical disorder. In Irene's case, she needed to take stock of her multiple sclerosis. And you? Sit down with a practitioner you trust and look at the list of causes for brain fog and mood disorders. Do not get a set of physicians who tell you what to do *or* tell you just what you want to hear. Get a balanced team approach. With the help of that team, you'll elucidate not just what the cause of your brain fog is and its appropriate treatments, but whether or not you need to pare down that laundry list of supplements, herbs, and medicines.

Once you've identified the cause of your brain fog, you can then focus on treating just the mood, using solutions from the earlier sections of this chapter. If you still have problems remaining with focus and attention, especially during hormonal events, you may want to read Chapter 5 on memory. If anxiety and trauma are the problem causing your brain fog, go on to Chapter 2 on anxiety. Finally, if you've ruled out all these causes and you find you're in the midst of a spiritual event that is disconnecting you from planet Earth, go to Chapter 6.

It can also be helpful to step away and take a meditational moment for yourself. There's a spiritual teacher named Baal Shem Tov who taught about the power of the self-imposed "exile." What is the self-imposed "exile"? You travel away from a familiar place, and you take only a few common objects. For some it's a long trip away from home. For others it's just a little jaunt. A spiritual journey in this way helps you deal with sadness and breeds humility. Such sabbaticals help you drive away distraction, focus on the emotion, and hear the voice of your soul. The self-imposed spiritual "exile" helps you in your mind to observe, describe, and allow. Not run away, not push away, not try to control, but simply allow the moment. Whether your depression comes from being angry about some events that you can't do anything about, or sadness or fear, taking a spiritual siesta helps you get spiritual clarity. And while you're in a self-imposed "exile," you realize you're not alone. In fact, while disconnected from the familiar, you get the opportunity of being connected with your higher power, God, or whatever you want to call it. You are with spirit. You are not alone.

THE AFFIRMATIONS

If you have brain fog that's increasing your chance toward depression and moodiness, look at it from the perspective of medical intuition. Brain fog often shreds the barrier between brain and body. In medical intuition, brain fog is a sixth-center issue. The sixth center has to do with perception and thought. If you have this cloudy mind, it impairs your capacity to see your way through a problem, and by definition you may have a sort of blindness toward it. Get a "Seeing Eye coach"; that is, get someone to help you see your way through your problem.

Here's another way to look at barriers in your mind: when you say an affirmation, does a negative thought come up? Whenever you say an affirmation and a negative thought pattern comes up, that's a barrier, and noticing that is great, because it's like doing a functional MRI. It lets you know that there is a thought pattern in your brain, a barrier, that's preventing you from changing. It gives you a chance to see what barriers are in the way of your healing.

Louise Hay has done extensive work on barriers and how to dissolve them. There are barriers in our lives to forgiveness, barriers in our lives to criticism, resentment, fear, and guilt. The most powerful affirmations for dissolving them are the following:

- I love and approve of myself.

- By choosing loving and joyous thoughts, I create a loving and joyous world. I am safe and free.

THE MESSAGE BEHIND THE MOOD

Whether you have problems with mind-body depression, moodiness, trauma, or brain fog, to maximize your healing, find the medical intuitive message behind the mood. Mood is a part of our body's intuitive guidance system that lets us know something needs to change. In the middle of the chaos, stop. Pull yourself out of whatever's happening. Like a seagull going above the sea, try to get another perspective. What is precipitating this mood? What have you lost? That's sadness. What is disrespecting you? That's anger. What do you think is threatening you? That's fear. And so on. If you can start the process of naming the emotion, you can learn how to respond to it effectively and then release it. By doing this process, which is actually the first step in dialectical behavioral therapy, you may stop the emotion in the brain from causing a domino effect and turning into a health problem in the body.

Chapter 2

ANXIETY

Has nervousness made it hard for you to feel comfortable around people? Has fear made it hard for you to use all your gifts, talents, and skills in education and work? Does worry prevent you from changing and growing and aging with confidence? If this is true, then anxiety is right now, this moment, affecting your brain and body.

For the last 30 years, during almost every consultation I've had, someone has always said, "Well, I'd do that if it weren't for the fear." I'd change my job, I'd go after a better relationship, I'd ask for a raise—it goes on. As Louise Hay says, "Without the fear, imagine the possibilities!" Whether you have always had chronic worry, whether you've had the long, slow burn of fear, whether you have had obsessions and compulsions and difficulty with control, whether you have had trauma in the past that makes you panicky and jumpy, or whether you have a terror of something life threatening, this chapter is for you.

WAYS OF LOOKING AT FEAR

Fear is an important part of our intuitive guidance system, protecting us from something we perceive as harmful. It prevents you from running into the middle of traffic or throwing caution to the wind. However, if fear holds you back from utilizing all your potential, you have a problem. If fear of rejection prevents you from meeting the love of your life, anxiety is keeping you from living fully. If fear of criticism and failure is preventing you from utilizing all of your career and intellectual gifts, then anxiety and worry are blocking your potential. And, finally, if you're afraid of being alone, you may find yourself stuck in a relationship that may in fact be abusive. On one hand, fear can protect us, but taken to the extreme, it can paralyze us.

BRAIN-BODY ANXIETY

Just like brain-body depression, brain-body anxiety is very common. We all know what it's like to emotionally feel nervous, panicky, uneasy, or worried. However, *body* anxiety is when your muscles get tense, your digestive tract feels bloated and stuck, you might feel like you have to go to the bathroom or you might get constipation. Sometimes you feel short of breath or your heart starts to race. You might feel that proverbial lump in your throat. You might have problems with paying attention; your mind might go blank. You might feel dizzy, have vertigo, and even feel like you're losing control.

Ultimately, we all know what it's like from time to time to shake with fear and be immobilized by terror. However, for about a third of us, panic and anxiety can escalate to the point where we have trouble leaving our houses (agoraphobia). Other people can avoid work promotions for fear of failure. And last but not least, some people have been traumatized in relationships, or in war, or their families have been so frightened or victimized, that they reexperience that fear in their current lives through shakiness, speechlessness, and numbness.

Louise Hay believes there's a choice between love and fear. Think about it. Love and fear? We experience fear with change, and we experience fear when we're not changing. Either way, we're gonna feel fear. We experience fear with the future, and we experience fear if we don't have a future. We experience fear when we take a chance, and we feel fear when we have no choice. We feel fear when we're alone, and we might feel overwhelmed with fear when we're in a crowd with too many people. Finally, we may be afraid of intimacy, but on the other hand, when our loved one leaves, we're afraid. Clearly, fear is part of the human experience. So, Louise Hay is right. We do have a choice between love and fear. But we need to know that love and fear go hand in hand. You can't have one without the other.

Love is the miracle we are all looking for. Not vanity. Not arrogance. But love. A great respect for ourselves and gratitude for the miracle of our bodies and our minds. Remind yourself, next time you are frightened, of this simple concept. Fear is not trusting yourself or loving yourself. And to put an additional spin on the issue, perhaps fear is an opportunity to employ faith. Faith in the divine, in the universe, or in a power outside yourself. Remind yourself of just these concepts the next time you are not feeling "good enough" and it's interfering with your ability to make a decision. (More about anxiety, faith, and spirituality in Chapter 6.)

ANXIETY AND MEDICAL INTUITION

In medical intuition, anxiety is part of your emotional guidance system that tells you something needs to change. In fact, anxiety is one of the most overly developed parts of your intuition. I have yet to meet anyone who was extremely intuitive who wasn't also very anxious. The amygdala, the area in the brain for intuition, is also the area for anxiety. So if you want to be intuitive, embrace, love, and honor that area of your brain that's twitchy and nervous. Susan Jeffers wrote a wonderful book called *Feel the Fear and Do It Anyway*. That book could have been named *Feel the Intuition and Do It Anyway*. You may feel fear when approaching something new in your life. When you feel something new and unfamiliar, when you feel something you think could threaten you, your adrenal gland produces epinephrine, that peppy neu-rotransmitter. For some individuals who are "prone" to that intu-itive anxious brain, stimulants like coffee push them over into panic and they become change-phobic. Susan Jeffers says that the real issue is not feeling the fear but how we hold the fear. Under-stand that change comes and goes. It's not static. And the fear along with the change can come and go. Intuition also comes and goes. You may sense that someone will call you, and then the phone rings, and then it's over with. You may sense something painful might happen to a loved one. It comes and it goes. To han-dle brain-body fear and anxiety is to learn how to handle change and intuition. How? We learn how to:

1. Feel the fear

2. Indicate what precipitated it

3. Respond to it effectively

4. Release it

Similarly, you might also name the intuition associated with the fear, name what precipitated it, respond to it effectively, and release it.

If you can't process fear and intuition effectively, it stops being a momentary thing. Instead, it will marinate, and it will create a daisy chain of symptoms in your brain and body. What was first fear or intuition then becomes nervousness, twitchiness, and a variety of other flavors of fear. Biochemical symptoms occur in your brain and body. Muscles tensing, lower back pain, nausea, butterflies in your stomach, constipation, diarrhea, shortness of breath, lump in your throat, problems with focus and attention (see Chapter 4), brain fog (see Chapter 1), clenching your teeth. All these are body symptoms of anxiety. They might also be body symptoms of an intuitive guidance system telling you that some-thing around you needs to be attended to.

How do you know that you have body anxiety? Let's go center by center. If you have fear and anxiety that stays "stuck on" in your brain-body, it creates a daisy chain of events, disrupts epinephrine and cortisol in your adrenal gland, affects your immune system and muscle contraction in your body, and increases your chance toward the following problems:

- First center: Eczema, hives, psoriasis, and rashes, indicating that you might have problems with feelings of safety and security in the world. Intuition letting you know there might be something wrong or a problem with someone in your family or another group in your life.

- Second center: Lower back pain, bladder problems, problems with libido, impotence, or unstable hormones, letting you know that you might be anxious about performing sexually or financially. It may also let you know intuitively that there's a problem in a relationship with a partner.

- Third center: Colitis, diarrhea, irritable bowel syndrome, nausea, ulcers, excessive eating, craving alcohol, unstable blood sugar, or loss of appetite may be letting you know that you feel criticized or anxious about work or your self-image. Alternatively, your intuition might be letting you know there's a problem with someone at work or in your environment who is criticizing you.

- Fourth center: Respiratory allergies like hay fever, shortness of breath, and asthma, as well as heart palpitations, may be letting you know that you have anxiety about speaking up in front of people when you feel criticized or rejected. Alternatively, your intuition may be picking up that someone near you might not feel safe and secure.

- Fifth center: A lump in the throat, grinding your teeth, sore throat, or hypothyroidism might let you know that you fear rejection and criticism if you were to speak.

- Sixth center: Dizziness, vertigo, insomnia, problems with attention and memory, letting you know you're insecure about the way you think or see the world.

- Seventh center: Problems with a life-threatening illness or aging in general.

All of these areas in your body are examples of brain-body anxiety, letting you know intuitively that fear has run amok in your life and that something needs to be paid attention to.

YOUR BRAIN ON FEAR

Louise, just like other mind-body practitioners and psychologists, sees the connection between fear, thoughts, and our experiences. There are many people who say we create the pain in our life. It's a little more complicated than that. As we said in the last chapter, if trauma shapes our brain to be drawn toward relationships and experiences that unwittingly duplicate our past trauma, then saying that we create the pain in our life may be only half the story. Me, being a neuroscientist and medical intuitive, I'm more likely to describe the phenomenon as the following: science shows us that like a moth to a flame, the biochemistry of the fear and memory areas in our brain is molded toward reenacting painful events in our life. Does that mean we are to blame for adversity? A better way to help ourselves heal our brains and our bodies to create health and happiness would be this: to identify how fear in our brain has corrupted brain circuits so that we might not be able to see healthier options, better opportunities to choose healthy friends, family, mates, education, and work. This chapter is about helping you heal the brain circuits for fear in your body and brain, whether you're predisposed to anxiety by genetics, trauma, or otherwise.

Now it is well known, whether to mind-body practitioners like Louise, psychologists, or brain scientists, that fearful thoughts perceive the environment in a fearful way and that increases our chance toward making less skillful choices within our families, relationships, finances, work, and so on. Part of fear is not knowing, and when you can allow yourself to learn the skills to manage fear, you can learn to thrive in the world of healthy families, relationships, finances, and so on.

As Louise has noted, we all hear things from our childhood on, the sounds of our parents, fearful voices warning us of danger. It's what we do with those sounds and those experiences that matters. If the people around you tell you to be afraid, if they tell you to experience life as always going to be unsafe, your thoughts will then tell you that the world is going to be a fearful place. And, yes, having a serious trauma—sexual abuse, incest, physical abuse in a marriage—will prime your brain and your body for fear and anxiety. You will be more likely to perceive the world, relationships, and families as fearful. However, we can change our thoughts, which will change how we see the world so we can make better choices in relationships and families and move away from re-creating our trauma and tragedy. You can't do anything about being caught in a flood, a typhoon, a war, or an environment where you are a refugee. You can't do anything about past sexual abuse, rape, or emotional or physical tragedy. And it's true that some of us believe we chose this life and we chose our parents and we chose these struggles we're experiencing. I'm simply trying to help all of us, within the life we're born into, learn to shape our brains and bodies so we can see the world as safer and more secure, so we can live with less fear.

THE FEAR NETWORK

How does science support healing your mind with meditation, affirmations, and intuition? To create wholeness in brain and body, we need to look at fear as a network. There is a fear network in our brain that is connected to vision, to hearing, and to our bodies and our health. There is a series of places in the brain that create fear. The primary area is the amygdala. All that we see, hear, smell, and taste gets funneled into the amygdala, especially what we've seen and heard from the past. There are two other brain areas that take the fear we experience in the amygdala and then make us act and think in a repetitive, compulsive fashion. One area is in the frontal lobe; it's called the anterior cingulate. The other area is called the caudate. You don't have to be a neuroanatomist to know that when you're anxious, you tend to have a gerbil wheel in your head that runs through your anxiety over and over again, and then you want to try to do something to change or control it, like checking the stove, making lists, cleaning your desk, and so on.

There are other areas in the brain that have to do with those thought patterns that make us feel more anxious or less. The frontal lobe area, the dorsolateral prefrontal cortex (DLPFC for short, if you want to impress your friends at a cocktail party), is the fourth area of the fear network. This area affects that aspect of fear in your thoughts that influences family, relationships, money, and work. So, you understand that by having fear in multiple areas of your brain, you have multiple capacities for resolving anxiety in your brain and your body. That's why solutions for anxiety aren't one size fits all.

The fifth area of the fear network is the orbital frontal area for empathy and bonding. This is the area that determines how trauma and anxiety affect your relationships. The sixth area, the insula, is the body area, where fear affects your health. Mind you, the insula connects to the adrenal gland, the area that governs the stress hormones cortisol and epinephrine. Yes, that's right, the adrenal gland stress response that's associated with adrenal fatigue. When you're fearful, when you have brain anxiety, you then get body anxiety. Your muscles tighten, your digestive tract tightens, you get constipation or diarrhea. Your bladder and vagina muscles tighten, causing uncomfortable sensations in both areas. Your heart races. You feel short of breath. It doesn't end there. You get the lump in the throat, the dizziness, the vertigo. Your mind races; you can't focus or pay attention.

Anxiety can affect any or all regions of this network, and like a telephone network, once it hits one region, it reverberates and can hit all of them. Something you see that's anxiety-provoking goes to the amygdala, and can then go to the insula, cause a body reaction, hit your adrenal gland, release cortisol, influence your immune system, and the next thing you know, within 24 to 48 hours, you have the flu. Or the epinephrine body reaction gives you a headache. And you'll say to someone, "Don't tell me that. You're giving me a headache."[1]

REWIRING THE NETWORK

So there you have the six brain areas of the fear network. Here's the thing: you can *rewire* this network. Just like a house that's been wired incorrectly for electricity, your brain can be rewired toward feeling safe and secure. By turning up the volume and intensity in any of these brain regions, you can alter how you see, hear, feel, and experience the world. You can change your thought patterns with affirmations via the dorsolateral prefrontal cortex, using statements like these:

> I release and let go of fears old and new. There is no longer any need for me to scare myself. I forgive all those who ever hurt me. I forgive myself for hurting others. I forgive myself for blaming and punishing myself. I forgive my parents for their fears and limitations. I now declare for myself that I am safe. I sleep and wake and move in complete safety.

You can do the same with cognitive behavioral therapy, dialectical behavioral therapy, or psychotherapy. You can also change the behavior that's wired in the caudate or anterior cingulate by working with a coach, a vocational counselor, and so on. You can work with a somatic therapist on your body memories. You can work with an immunologist and nutritionist on that adrenal fatigue / adrenal gland / cortisol pattern. You may have been terrorized or traumatized in the past. You may have had fear in your life then. But you can create a world in your brain and your body that's safe, peaceful, and secure.

Then there's medicine: with it, we can learn to turn up the volume or turn down the pitch of any of these brain areas with supplements, medicines, or other treatments. Traditional psychiatry uses SSRIs like Lexapro or Zoloft to treat anxiety. We may also use alternative remedies like 5-HTP, rhodiola, GABA, valerian, kava kava, passion flower, lemon balm, magnesium, and others (see details in the All Is Well Clinic).

Traditional psychiatry has supported psychotherapy or psychoanalysis that helps you develop a supportive relationship with a therapist. Louise Hay helps you use affirmations to do "loving the inner child" exercises where you learn to re-parent yourself. Either or both of these practices can help you rewire your brain away from fear and toward promoting a more loving, less fearful world. Can these practices really change the structure of those six areas in our brain network? In fact, the science of epigenetics says they can. Yes, early emotional trauma alters your brain circuits, creating changes in the memory areas of the amygdala and hippocampus; however, those cells in your hippocampus grow and give birth to new ones just like you can grow and give birth to a new you. We can't change the past, but we can create a new future.[2]

How to Switch Your Brain from Fear to Safety

First, don't use the words *stressed* or *overwhelmed*, because when you say "stressed" or "overwhelmed," you don't know you're actually anxious. Those words aren't going to help you heal your brain circuits for fear. If anything, they just keep the nervousness reverberating within your brain and your body. For decades, people have lumped anxiety, nervousness, and panic together under the blanket term *stress*. I'm so stressed! You're so stressed! I'm worried! I'm nervous! There's so much stress at work! So, then, we have stress-reduction exercises. You sit in a position, you breathe, you say, "I'm reducing my stress." Then you go back to work, and you get panic-stricken, only to return to the pose of "I'm breathing and releasing my stress." Only to go back into the workplace and get panic-stricken again! Then you go home, and you worry about work. Back to the relaxing space.

Are we unstressed yet? No, we're not! Because we haven't named the emotion, the fear or anxiety, so we can respond to it effectively, and then release it. As Dr. Phil says, "If you can't name it, you can't fix it." So if you say, "I'm nervous," you can then look around and say, "Why am I nervous?" And then you'll get a thought pattern. *Oh, it's because I think I'm gonna fail.* And that's in your frontal lobe. You then get to look around the fear network to see where the emotion and thought is coming from, and only then can you learn to change the thought so that you can release the feeling and move on.

After you've gotten rid of words from your vocabulary like *stress* and *overwhelmed*, look into discontinuing the use of the terms *out of sorts* and *overcome*. While you're at it, eliminate *nervous breakdown* too. After a three-year psychiatry residency, I still don't know what a nervous breakdown is.

Now that we've gotten rid of words that make it hard to identify the emotion—fear—let's work on thought patterns that help us all marinate in nervousness and worry. Eliminate the word *should*. *Woulda, coulda, shoulda* are self-blame words that are embedded in your frontal lobe that make you worried and tense. As if you didn't feel disempowered enough, criticized enough, there you are saying, "Well, you know, I should have done this." Not only are they criticizing you; you're criticizing you too. As Louise says, "*Should* is a word that makes us prisoners." And, as a result, that thought in your frontal lobe just makes you more fearful. Louise says to change the "should" into "could." I like that. Cognitive behavioral therapy would like that. Why? Because *should* tells you what you did wrong in the past. *Could* is something that you can look forward to changing. It's more empowering. And so, now is your opportunity to perform a radical "worry-word-ectomy" on all the vocabulary that's disempowering, self-criticizing, and paralyzing you from moving forward and changing. In the next chapter, on addiction, you'll get an opportunity to remove shame and blame words as well. There is an intricate connection between anxiety, shame, and addiction.

THE ALL IS WELL CLINIC

The rest of this chapter is devoted to the All Is Well Clinic, where you get a virtual experience of how to heal your anxiety, worry, and panic.

I. CHRONIC WORRY

Has your brain become a prisoner to worry? Look at the list of symptoms here and find out which apply to you.

MIND SYMPTOMS

- You feel fear, worry, anxiety, and apprehension about your family, relationships, work, or children.

- Your fears about nearly every area of your life tend to consume your thoughts and feelings.

- You have been nervous, anxious, and worried since an early age, and it's hard for you to remember a time when you didn't worry.

- You have problems with irritability and moodiness.

- You also suffer from hard-to-treat depression.

BODY SYMPTOMS

- Your muscles are tight, and often it makes your joints ache.

- You get easily exhausted.

- You feel restless, keyed up, and jumpy most of the time.

- Sleep has been a perennial issue. Either you have problems falling asleep or staying asleep, or you have unrestful sleep.

- You have trouble focusing and paying attention.

- Your mind often goes blank.

- You have problems with allergies.

- You have problems with eczema and psoriasis.

- You have problems with nausea, heartburn, and IBS.

- You experience urinary urgency and/or frequency.

- You have hypothyroidism.

- You experience dizziness or vertigo.

- Your blood pressure is unstable.

- Your hair is thinning.

If this sounds like you, chronic worry may be preventing you from having the healthiest, happiest life you can experience. Read on to the following case.

ADELE: WORRY, WORRY, WORRY

Adele came to me because, well, she was always worrying.

THE INTUITIVE READING

When I first started to read Adele, her mind swirled with a sense of failure about her life or everyone else's life. All I could see were thoughts about catastrophes, whether it was in her family, finance, work, everywhere.

THE BODY

Adele's mind was a buzz of thoughts and activity, so much that it seemed that she couldn't focus or pay attention. The muscles felt tight in her neck like rubber bands, making for bandlike pressure around her head. The muscles in her colon seemed tight as well. Did she have trouble going to the bathroom, having regular bowel movements? Then there was the lower back, the joints. Muscle tightness seemed to be in every joint in her body. Her sciatic area, her wrists, all of her joints seemed like they were in a vise. Finally,

I wondered how Adele could get to sleep with all those bees buzzing in her head.

THE FACTS

Adele said that for as long as she could remember, people had called her a worrywart. She worried about her parents, their marriage, their finances. She worried about getting into a good school. Then she worried about whether she could get into a good college. She worried about politics, the economy. Later, she worried about her daughter, Barbara, and her family. Worry, worry, worry. In fact, much of her mind was so taken up by worrying about future catastrophes that she had trouble focusing on anything else. Let's add up the diagnoses that Adele got to worry about. She was told by doctors that she had:

1. ADHD
2. Tension headaches, possibly migraines
3. Depression
4. Anxiety
5. IBS
6. Lower back pain
7. Generalized anxiety disorder

THE SOLUTION

If you, like Adele, are worrying, how does that lead to all those symptoms? How do you get all these physical problems with anxiety? Like depression, where there's body depression and brain depression, anxiety has the same format. We can see brain and body anxiety as well. When the amygdala starts to spike out anxious signals, all six members of the fear network start to reverberate nervousness, and, as you remember, the signal gets sent down to the adrenal gland. The adrenal gland creates epinephrine, which makes all the muscles in your body tend to tighten. That accounts for headaches, joint pain, and, over time, exhaustion. The tight muscles also change the peristalsis in your bowel and increase your chance toward constipation and IBS. The epinephrine disrupts your capacity to focus, pay attention, and ultimately remember things. Thus, you may be diagnosed with ADHD. The chronic anxiety increases your chance for fatigue, adrenal fatigue, and chronic fatigue syndrome. Needless to say, all that exhaustion during the day and that over-adrenalated epinephrine from the adrenal gland makes it hard for you to fall asleep at night, thus, the insomnia.

THE TREATMENTS

If you, like the vast majority of people, suffer from chronic anxiety and worry, you may have learned it's not easy to get rid of. You'll try a medicine, nutritional supplement, herb, or acupuncture or other treatment. After a month, you may get some relief, but two months later the worry and panic come back with a vengeance. Why? I remember when I was in medical school, back in the olden days, the primary medicines for anxiety were Valium, Xanax, and Klonopin, medicines that tend to work at a specific dosage for a month or two and then stop working. I might add, these medicines, benzodiazepines, are highly addictive. I remember I asked one of my teachers how long people were supposed to stay on these medicines, and he said, "As long as the person feels anxious." The problem with anxiety and worry is that the brain deals with fear like a shell game. If you have one treatment that addresses one area of the fear network, the other areas somehow compensate, and a month or two later your anxiety is back. In the old days, doctors would just raise the dosage of the medicine and you'd end up getting addicted to more and more meds that eventually would stop working. I'm thrilled, and you will be too, that people don't have their anxiety treated that way anymore.

Why is anxiety such a cagey or slippery symptom to nail down and get rid of? Fear is a fundamental part of how your brain and body are structured. You'll learn later on in this chapter that many people who tend toward nervousness and anxiety are more likely to have exaggerated intuitive gifts. It's impossible to keep the intuitive gifts and get rid of the anxiety entirely. So, many people who are very intuitive, porous, or sensitive also struggle with lifelong anxiety. If this is you, you'll learn how to capture the intuitive gifts and soothe the edginess and worry that accompany this brain style. If you suffer from worry, you need to learn how to soothe the chronic anxiety that reverberates in the fear circuits in your brain.

- First, consider dialectical behavioral therapy and/or cognitive behavioral therapy. Dialectical behavioral therapy specifically is a class that will teach you how to regulate your anxious mind and body. Consider it a class like driver's ed that teaches you how to operate your unique edgy, tense brain.

- Consider various body treatments that can reduce the keyed-up chronic adrenalation that your mind-body fear network creates. Regular daily exercise, 30 to 45 minutes at least five days a week, releases opiates that can calm, distract, and transform your worry. Massage increases serotonin from one area of your fear network. The added benefit of this treatment is that it can help with muscle pain. Yoga is another movement practice that with deep breathing exercises and relaxation can profoundly improve anxiety and worry. Yoga also helps with breathing and blood pressure irregularities that tend to occur with chronic worry.

- Meditation can help discipline your mind to help you stop or control your worried thoughts. Many of the exercises you'll learn in dialectical behavioral therapy are in fact based on mindfulness meditation.

- Consider a hobby—anything that involves a repetitive task. An activity like knitting or woodworking, especially if it requires the same movement over and over again, engages part of your fear network to release GABA, a calming neurotransmitter. Akin to rocking a baby, when we do some mindless, repetitive, cyclic task, it disengages our mind and seemingly puts us in another realm, and for the moment, disconnects us from our worry.

- Repetitive prayers or chants evoke the part of the brain, the caudate, that releases GABA. In addition to the pharmacology of prayer, when you set aside regular time for contact with the divine or a greater power, you are exercising faith, which is, in a way, the universal antidote to anxiety and worry.

THE MEDICINES

While you're learning how to rewire worry and anxiety that chronically reverberate in your brain and body, you may want to use nutritional supplements, herbs, and medicines.

- Taking 5-HTP, 100 milligrams three times a day, can hit the same serotonin receptor as those SSRIs like Lexapro, Paxil, and Effexor do, and 5-HTP doesn't give you sexual side effects. Rhodiola is also antianxiety, and it buffers your body's anxious tendency toward cortisol problems. And, finally, ashwagandha is also excellent, like rhodiola, for brain and body anxiety.

- There are some nutritional supplements, helpful alternatives for generalized anxiety disorder. Passion flower and lemon balm especially can be very helpful. Check your nearest holistic health food store for tinctures or other supplements, but consider avoiding valerian or kava kava. They tend to stop working after two weeks. You might be thrilled to know that lemon balm can also help with chronic fatigue and fibromyalgia that's associated with Epstein-Barr virus and Lyme because it has antiviral and antibacterial qualities. And both herbs are very helpful for insomnia and digestive problems.

- Gingko biloba goes after the benzodiazepine receptor, the same receptor that Klonopin, Valium, and Xanax do, that we talked about earlier. However, it's not addictive like those medicines, and it also helps with focus and attention, which many people with anxiety tend to have problems with. Be careful, though; it's a blood thinner. Ask your doctor if it's safe for you.

- There are several types of ginseng that may be helpful. Asian ginseng and Siberian ginseng are two of these. The ginsengs are specifically good for brain anxiety and body anxiety because they buffer cortisol that may impact your capacity to have a healthy immune system. The ginsengs also sharpen your attention and memory and help you get to sleep, all of which tend to be problematic when you have anxiety.

- The next class of medicines is antidepressants. You can take Lexapro, Paxil, Effexor, and other SSRIs for anxiety. However, they're not very helpful for chronic worry. Many people gain weight and have sexual side effects. And, by the way, you might want to minimize the alcohol too, because, just like benzodiazepines, alcohol tends to hit the same GABA receptor and combat anxiety, not to mention insomnia. At first, you'll feel great with the alcohol. *I'm not nervous anymore. What, me worry?* However, again, you'll have two worries, not one. One, you'll be anxious in the morning, as well as possibly having brain fog, and two, you'll end up having an increased susceptibility for addiction. There has to be another way. (See Chapter 3.)

THE AFFIRMATIONS

So, let's just say you've set aside your alcohol and your Valium, and you've considered 5-HTP or rhodiola, Gingko biloba, and ginseng. Is that it? Are you now going to be not nervous? No, it may take a while to rewire the thought patterns in your brain. In addition to cognitive behavioral therapy and dialectical behavioral therapy, affirmations can have a prolonged effect on changing particularly entrenched anxiety-provoking thoughts and worries. When you keep replaying worried thoughts you've been learning since childhood, it makes anxiety even more entrenched in your brain and body. Affirmations are a particularly potent way to change entrenched thoughts from fear to safety. Louise helps us with affirmations like these:

Begin to take a deep breath, and as you exhale, let your fear out. Imagine that every time you exhale now, you are releasing old fears, some a little at a time and some all at once in a big, big exhale. Now, affirm and declare, "I release and I let go. I let go of fears old and new. There is no longer any need to scare myself. I forgive all those who have ever hurt me. I forgive myself for hurting others. I forgive myself for blaming and punishing myself. I forgive my parents for their fears and limitations, and I now declare for myself that I am safe. I sleep and wake and move in complete safety.

I now create a reality for myself of oneness and security. I create an island of safety around me. I can see this island in my mind's eye. It is safe and serene. It is beautiful and green. I walk freely everywhere on this island in perfect peace. This island becomes my world, and everyone in this island enjoys the same safety. We are all peaceful. Everyone in my world is peaceful. I am safe. I am secure. I am at peace. Every corner of my world is a safe place. I am safe in the daytime. I am safe at night. I walk in peace. My inner intelligence always leads me in the peaceful byways. My bed is a safe place. I release the day with love and I embrace sleep. I am safe when I am asleep. I am safe during the night. My dreams are dreams of joy. I awaken feeling safe and secure. I enter the new day with joyous anticipation, for it is a day that has never been lived before. I know and affirm that I am safe in this new day.

I am always safe in my home and all who enter my home do so in safety and peace. My food is safe and healthful and nourishing. Any room in my dwelling place is safe and peaceful. My home is a peaceful shelter. I am relaxed at home. I radiate love wherever I am. I surround myself with loving people. Only love goes from me, and only love comes back to me. I forgive others and move on. I am forgiven and I am free.

All forms of transportation I use are safe. I am safe in cars and buses, in trains and planes, even on bicycles and skateboards, no matter what form of transportation I use, I am safe and secure. I am able to relax when traveling. I am a peaceful traveler.

I know I am safe at work. I work in a place that is harmonious. I love the work that I do. I am safe with my co-workers. I am safe with my boss. My job is safe and mine as long as I want it. I am relaxed and peaceful when I am working. Even when working to a deadline, I feel peaceful, and the more peaceful I am, the more efficient I am. I do my best work when I relax. I create a relaxed, joyful atmosphere wherever I am. My boss appreciates and loves the way I work. I am calm and secure at all times.

Wherever I go in this world, I take my island of safety with me. This island of safety also protects my family. Every member of my family is safe and protected. I release all worries about my family. I surround every member of my family in thoughts of safety and peace.

The dark is my friend. The dark is comforting to me. I move through the dark with ease. I am safe in the dark. There is nothing in the dark for me to fear. I am always safe and well protected. From the smallest to the largest, from the youngest to the oldest, from home to school to work to play and home again, everyone is moving through life in peace and harmony. I free my family to be who they are, and to live life in their own way, knowing that no harm can befall them. My family also allows me to be who I am and to live my life in the way I think is best. We are all safe and free. I relax in the knowledge that I am at peace.

I feel safe and secure in my spiritual beliefs. I feel at one with my creator. I know that my creator has only my joy and my well-being in mind. I trust in the power that created me to protect me at all times and under all circumstances. I was created to be all that I can be; I am safe with love. All my lessons are easily learned. I easily release that which no longer works. It is safe for me to learn. I approach new lessons with joyous anticipation. It is easy for me to learn. I am willing to learn. I love to learn new things. Life gives me easy lessons."

Finally, in addition to affirmations, consider cognitive behavioral therapy and dialectical behavioral therapy to rewire the thought patterns in your dorsolateral prefrontal cortex, those words that reverberate in your brain and disrupt your biochemistry toward panic and away from serenity.

II. Obsessive and Compulsive Anxiety

Now, when it comes to obsessions and compulsions, do you tend to have this brand of anxiety? Take a look at the list of symptoms here that you may experience in addition to the ones we saw in the previous section.

Mind Symptoms

- Repetitive images: an anxiety-provoking picture that you can't get out of your mind intrudes during your day, whether you're talking with someone, driving, or whatever.

- Circular thought: a thought, like a broken record, keeps going around in your mind. *I've got to do [blank]. I've got to check the [blank]. I've got to clean the [blank].*

- Continuous and systematic action: you actually have to carry out that thought repeatedly. You do [blank], check the [blank], clean the [blank], over and over again.

- Like weeds in a garden, these images, thoughts, or actions take over your mind, consuming your day and making it harder for you to have normal relationships, productive work, or peace of mind.

- Your mind is focused on details, rules, lists, order, and organization, so much that people often note you miss the point of a project.

- You are perfectionistic to a fault, compelled to erase every flaw from a task. However, sometimes it makes it hard for you to tolerate a lack of perfectionism in others.

- It's easier for you to bear down on productivity at work. However, sometimes that tends to displace time in your schedule for friendship and leisure activities.

Body Symptoms

In addition to the symptoms in the previous section, you may have these:

- Your muscles are extremely tight.

- You have a forward-bent posture.

- You have digestive allergies, IBS, and/or constipation.

If this sounds like you, don't worry. With your obsessiveness and compulsivity and drive to get it right, you can fix your obsessive-compulsive anxious tendency if you put your mind to it. Read on to the following case. Remember, you're in the virtual All Is Well Clinic. We have the technology. We can help you.

Beth and Charles: Obsessions and Compulsions

Beth, 43, called the All Is Well Clinic because she was concerned about her husband, Charles, 43. She thought he might be a "control fanatic."

THE INTUITIVE READING

When I first read Charles, it felt like he was an "emperor." Emperors rule the kingdom. Their way of loving people is to make decisions for them, handle everything for them. That may feel great if you want everything taken care of. However, after a while, you may end up feeling that your freedom is being impinged just a little bit. And I sensed that when people around Charles tried to strike out in independence, he got annoyed. Unless you did things his way, he'd get annoyed. Everything at home had to be his way. People had to fit into his order. Otherwise, he got nervous and then angry. I could sense that Charles didn't like change.

THE BODY

Looking at Charles's body, it felt like all the muscles were tight as a rock. Every muscle fixed in position. Braced at attention, like a Marine at inspection. Other than minor digestion and skin problems, I didn't think he'd ever admit to any physical symptoms.

THE FACTS

Beth said that yes, indeed, it was in fact true that Charles had trouble with change. He had obsessiveness. He had compulsiveness. Everyone called him a control fanatic. At home, their kitchen drawers, their closets, even their garage was a masterpiece of perfect organization, order, and control. And if anyone tried to move anything, there was a price to pay. The same was true at Charles's work. When someone at home or at work tried to suggest a change of any kind—from a renovation project to a new piece of furniture to a new way of thinking—Charles would snap unless people submitted to his way of doing things. Beth wanted to know if supplements, medicines, or other remedies would help with his symptoms.

THE SOLUTION

Every family, every company, needs someone who's obsessive and compulsive to help everybody stay in line and help the system run well. However, if you are that person who is very organized, very perfectionistic, but tends to be obsessive and compulsive and, at the extreme, can't get those repetitive images and thoughts out of your mind, your compulsion is going to take over your life.

When you get nervous, do you try to order your environment? When you're insecure, and the world around you is changing, do you try to clean your desktop, clean out your purse, or make lists and schedules? If a lot of order and perfection helps reduce your anxiety, this can make you great as an accountant or some other kind of detail-oriented professional. However, if your perfectionism and order spill over onto the people around you, then you will begin to have problems. People might think of you as a control fanatic. Then you're going to feel misunderstood and underappreciated. They may think you are "rigid," overly organized, inflexible, when really all you're trying to do is help.

I have a friend who is a fabulous secretary. She is the epitome of efficiency. However, she is very nervous. Everything in her life looks like it's calibrated with a protractor, and to be a little bit of an imp, when she went to the ladies' room once, I sneaked into her office and I changed just a degree, a millimeter, the things on her desk. And then when she came back from the bathroom, I watched as she glanced at her desktop and put everything, millimeter by millimeter, back in its place. Because otherwise, it was just too anxiety-provoking for her. It was clear that the woman used her environmental control as Valium.

Do you order your environment as if it were Xanax? And if you can't control your schedule and if there are out-of-control events around you, too much change, do you get panic-stricken? If this is you (and I must add, a little bit of me too), then your anxiety may come out in the form of obsessions and compulsions. If you don't do these perfectionistic things in your environment, you may be haunted by images and thoughts of what will happen if you don't.

You are going to be loved for your neatness. People will call you and ask you if you have Virgo somewhere in your chart. They will want you to make the plans for the trip or help them pack. However, there is a chance that you might drive yourself and others just a little bit crazy and it might take you too long at times to finish up your projects at work, because, like weeds in the garden, obsessions and compulsions in your frontal lobe can take over your emotions, the space in your house, and the space in your life. Not to mention the fact that your need to keep your life under tight control can become memorialized in tight control in the muscles in your body. You might find yourself having lower back pain, shoulder pain, neck pain, headaches, and the like.

THE TREATMENTS

People with this form of anxiety often don't want to take medicines, supplements, or herbs. Their symptoms of obsessiveness and compulsivity make it difficult for them to take pills into their body. Perhaps it's the excessive norepinephrine that makes them jittery? Perhaps it's the thought that they can control the problem on their own without taking anything? Or the uncertainty of not knowing which of the long lists of side effects they see on the Internet could happen to them? If this is you, you may want to try the solutions for anxiety—medicines, supplements, herbs—that we saw in the previous section, but start with one-half or one-quarter of the dose. Before you take the medicine/supplement/herb, look in the mirror and say to yourself, "This is such a low dose, it will have no effect *and* it will have no side effect." By conditioning your brain and body in this way, you are talking to your mind centers distributed in every tissue in your body, telling them you can be safe accepting help from something outside of you. You may also want to have a coach or therapist help you with dialectical behavioral therapy, cognitive behavioral therapy, or mindfulness to help you learn to reorganize the emotional and thought patterns in your brain and body.

In addition, try antianxiety supplements—HTP, rhodiola, or ashwagandha—or medicines such as Zoloft, Paxil, or others if they don't cause you side effects. Use yoga or massage to relax those stiff, tight, boardlike muscles. Yamuna body rolling, or other modalities that help bring awareness to your muscles, might help loosen the muscles creating tension in the tendons and the fascia. The Alexander Technique may help you bring consciousness to your posture, which can tend to buckle forward with the muscle tension. There are other things you can try as well. Ask your nearby holistic health care practitioner for essential oils that might be helpful for calming, relaxing, and soothing you.

THE AFFIRMATIONS

Now for the affirmations that will help create more flexibility in your brain and reduce anxiety, obsessions, and compulsions.

The affirmation Louise offers for this situation is:

> Relationships are safe for me. All my relationships are loving. It is safe for me to be open and honest in a relationship, and I allow others to be open and honest with me. It is safe for me to love. It is safe for me to take care of myself in a relationship. It is safe for me to be myself with others. It is safe for me to learn and grow. I am willing to change. I am willing to become more of who I am. It is safe for me to be all that I can be. I threaten no one when I am myself, and all of my relationships support me in my growth. I am safe with my friends. I am safe with my acquaintances. I am safe with the public. I am even safe with my so-called enemies. I now attract only loving people into my life. I am safe at every age.

Relying on your cognitive behavioral therapy, dialectical behavioral therapy, affirmations, and any supplements and medicines you're taking, you'll start to rewire the thought patterns in your frontal lobe and your fear pathways. You will learn to sail forward with a true rhythm of life, just a little bit less in control.

III. TRAUMA AND MIND-BODY ANXIETY

Have you experienced an event or events in your life that were so traumatic they were outside the realm of normal experience—events such as rape, incest, abuse, witnessing a murder, or the loss of your body's physical integrity? If so, trauma may have shaped your mind and body toward anxiety, just as you read in Chapter 1 that it can shape your mind and body toward depression.

In addition to the symptoms we outlined in the previous two sections, look at the lists below and check off the items that apply to your life right now.

MIND SYMPTOMS

- You experienced painful emotional or physical trauma in your family growing up.

- You've suffered emotional or physical trauma in one or more of your relationships.

- There has been an event in your life in which you've been threatened with such serious physical or emotional harm that it would be out of the range of what we consider normal life experience. Some examples might be living through war, witnessing an accident with loss of life or limb, experiencing rape or incest, or seeing your children suffer abuse.

- Whatever the trauma you've experienced, you tend to have "repeat performances" of this painful pattern in one relationship after another, one job after another, and so on. The painful pattern seems to replay over and over in your life like the movie *Groundhog Day*.

- You have thought patterns of terror, fright, panic, and edginess.

- You have a feeling that you might be hurt or harmed, or that someone might reject or criticize you.

- You believe you won't get the help you need.

- You feel you're incompetent to change the situation.

- You feel like you're going crazy.

BODY SYMPTOMS

In addition to the symptoms in the previous section, you may have these:

- Trembling and shaking

- Hot flashes and cold chills

- Numbness and tingling

- Nausea or a sick feeling in your stomach

- Pressure in your chest

- A pounding heart

- Cold sweats

- Shortness of breath

- A lump in your throat

- Dizziness and vertigo

- Feeling like you're "out of your body"

- Feeling like you're dying

In every chapter in this book, you'll find that trauma can rewire the brain in some area of function. But don't worry—we have solutions in the All Is Well Clinic. If this describes you, read on. As a client in this virtual clinic, you will have a whole host of solutions you can use with your health care team to create physical relief and emotional serenity.

DOLLY: ANXIETY AFTER A TRAUMATIC EXPERIENCE

Dolly, 28, came to me because her family was concerned for her after a traumatic childhood.

THE INTUITIVE READING

I saw Dolly as if she were in a house and someone was walking in and out and slamming the door. The individual in the house who seemed to be creating terror seemed to have violent mood swings, so potent that they would affect people nearby, in the same room or even on other floors of the house. It felt like Dolly's world was threatened, and the horror of being around this person reverberated in her body. After meeting that family, I saw that Dolly's life seemed unstable in so many realms. Did she have a hard time making friends outside of her family? I had a hard time seeing a partner or other relationships. It didn't seem like she could last in a job and make enough money to support herself.

THE BODY

Her head felt shaky. Her body felt shaky. Everything about Dolly's mind and body felt nervous. Was there dizziness and vertigo in her head? I sensed a lump in her throat. It seemed that she was constantly out of breath, and her heart skipped a beat in a way that was terrifying. I could see that her digestive tract tended to look like it had butterflies in it, giving her that nauseous feeling. All the muscles in her body seemed tight, making her feel exhausted. I could see Dolly up all hours of the night trying to get to sleep.

THE FACTS

It turned out that Dolly had seen her father beat her mother on multiple occasions. His explosive temper drove away everyone except, of course, Dolly. Dolly still lived with her father because she couldn't manage to find Mr. Right, nor could she make any job last. Her problems with focus and attention made it hard for her to finish school, and she was soon diagnosed with attention deficit hyperactivity disorder (ADHD). Dolly told me that doctors gave her antidepressants for irritability, and then they said she had bipolar disorder, the idea of which she thought was ridiculous. Dolly began to medicate away the memories of her father's violence with alcohol and marijuana. All she wanted was to have the episodes of panic go away. She wanted the chest pounding, the choking, the trembling, the nausea all to just leave so she could start to have a happy life.

THE SOLUTION

Many of us have events in our life that are traumatic. A parent dies when we're in middle age. One of our children gets a minor illness and we're terrified that they may not survive. A child may be diagnosed with a learning disability, or we may have a fender bender on the highway. All of us have the resilience in our brains and bodies to bounce back; however, when we experience an event that is over the top in magnitude, such as up-close, personal experience of war, watching a loved one die, being a victim of rape or abuse, and so on, the horrific memories get laid down in our brains and bodies. Psychiatry names this post-traumatic stress disorder (PTSD). The most recent studies with brain scans indicate that in PTSD sufferers, the fear network is not working properly. Whether it's revealed by PET scans or magnetic spectroscopy, we know that the elements of the network produce aberrant amounts of serotonin, GABA, or other neurotransmitters.[3]

If you, like the person in this case, have had serious trauma in your life, you may suffer from anxiety as well as depression and from its effects in your brain and body. First, understand that part of all life is distress. From the moment we're born, we cry. It's painful. Daily all of us have one event or another that causes distress. Some amount of "stress," pain, is necessary for us to grow and develop. Some even believe that crisis is necessary to challenge us and force us forward to accomplish greater and greater feats. Whether it's taking our first steps or the anxiety we face on the first day of kindergarten or the first day of college, all of us have to face normal amounts of fear and other feelings so we can recruit other brain regions to adjust our thoughts and move on to the next life mission. However, if we've been threatened or someone close to us has been threatened with bodily harm or sexual violence, this can be considered PTSD if four basic symptoms continue longer than a month:

1. You keep having reverberating memories of the event in the form of dreams, images, or body reactions.

2. You go out of your way to avoid situations that remind you of the event. This might be avoiding a highway or highways around it after you've had a car accident, or avoiding the sounds of airports if

you've seen a helicopter crash, and so on. You avoid situations where you hear, see, or sense reminders of the trauma.

3. You have changes in how your thoughts work, your mood functions, and your body functions after the event. Your memory is like a fog. You can't remember events. You may feel like you're out of your body, you dissociate, and as a result you may have a distorted memory of events. You may either blame yourself or you blame the world. You may start to withdraw from activities. You may feel numb or detached from loved ones. And somehow, that overall dulling in your brain makes it hard for you to experience love, joy, and satisfaction.

4. Last but not least, your body remains keyed up after the trauma with norepinephrine, that adrenal gland stress hormone, which causes you to be jumpy, reactive, and hypervigilant; your muscles will tighten, and you'll get exhausted. This also makes it hard for you to focus, pay attention, and, yes, fall asleep. Your jumpiness and moodiness may make you more likely to have anger outbursts, causing problems with your relationships, your job, or your functioning as a whole.

The symptoms of panic with PTSD are not the most paralyzing consequence. What is the most paralyzing consequence is you restrict your life. You start to avoid things that remind you of the trauma. The circle of avoidance gets greater and greater and greater and greater. Those highways you started to avoid after the accident start to become back roads as well, until you stop driving completely. Hearing traffic noises may bother you, at which time you start closing the windows in your house and just don't want to listen to any kind of car at all. You may stay home more and more. When people start to tell you, "Hey, listen, you're getting more and more restricted in your life," you'll say, "Well, I could do more, but I'd rather not." You start to think, *What would happen if? Well, I could go in a car, but what if an accident happens?* A minority of people, 5 percent, actually end up unable to leave their homes, a homebound situation called agoraphobia.

THE TREATMENTS

If you have suffered from a serious trauma in your life that affects your mind and body, go to Chapter 1 and read section III in the All Is Well Clinic there. Chances are your trauma increases your chance toward depression, and many of the solutions in that section may apply to you. Those solutions can help you support your brain and body as you heal the past and create a healthier mind-body for greater happiness in the present and the future.

And when it comes to suffering from panic after a trauma, it's important to look at all the medical conditions that could make your anxiety, nervousness, and twitchiness worse. Have a physician check out your thyroid, your blood sugar, your calcium, and your adrenal gland. Hyperthyroidism, Cushing's syndrome (excessive cortisol or adrenal gland exhaustion), and a parathyroid gland problem can all mimic or worsen panic attacks. Go to a cardiologist and have an EKG to check out your heart rhythm. If you have symptoms of dizziness, vertigo, and feeling "out of your body," go to a neurologist to make sure you aren't also having a brain wave problem. Go to an ear, nose, and throat doctor to make sure your middle ear isn't also causing some symptom. Notice I'm not saying that if you treat these physical health problems, your panic will completely go away. Traumatic experience may increase your chance toward having all of these disorders, so it's important to treat both the physical problems and the emotional distress. While you're at it, make sure that your shortness of breath isn't made worse by allergies or asthma.

Have a trusted coach, counselor, or nutritionist go over your diet to make sure that medicine, supplements, or foods aren't making your panic worse, especially caffeine and alcohol, not to mention cocaine and marijuana. You might say, "Marijuana? How could that possibly make my panic worse?" Well, it may make you calm at first, but over time it will make your brain foggier in terms of attention and memory. It's called "borrowing from Peter to pay Paul." Using marijuana may calm your nerves but mess up your attention; using alcohol can help you fall asleep, but you'll end up feeling more depressed. It's important to work with a trusted practitioner to balance your psychopharmacology so that the things you're doing to self-medicate your panic aren't making your brain and body worse.

Other solutions? Now that you have been medicinally and pharmacologically rewiring your body, you might as well do the same with your brain and your behavior. Cognitive behavioral therapy can help you start to identify the thought patterns in your brain, the "what if" and "I could, but I'd rather not" thought patterns. Exposure therapy can help stop the pattern in which you avoid more and more things in the world. This is a procedure where you use imagery and with a tremendous amount of support start to imagine past traumatic events and conceive present circumstances that remind you of them. With support, you'll learn to desensitize your brain and body.[4]

It's important, at this stage of your treatment, to tell yourself that you are a brave survivor for having come so far and that you want, paradoxically, to face new situations that might be scary and out of your comfort zone. Holding two thought patterns that are seemingly opposite concepts (i.e., paradox) is the key to healing trauma. For example, "I love myself just the way I am" is a phrase that can be coupled with its seeming opposite, "I want to change." Often people who have a history of trauma and abuse have difficulty holding paradox and are prone to black-and-white thinking. So, you might say, "I'm a survivor, I've come this far, this is what I learned to do to feel safe." However, if the way you've learned to feel safe is by limiting your life to only one or two friends, you'll feel less anxiety at first, but in the long run you'll socially starve. Limiting happiness and freedom because you are panic-stricken means you are still shackled to your trauma. That's all right. You can love yourself where you are *and* want more.

How do you do that? Dialetical behavioral therapy helps you train your mind to handle seemingly opposite thoughts and get rid of the black-and-white thinking that escalates panic and limits your life. Dialectical behavioral therapy for many is the treatment of choice for PTSD and panic disorder. This kind of cognitive behavioral therapy is based on Tibetan Buddhism and mindfulness. It helps you learn how to regulate panic, fear, sadness, anger, shame, and guilt. You may also want to consider hypnotherapy, EMDR (stands for "eye movement desensitization and reprocessing"), and other therapies that help people alter their mind-body networks for trauma.

OTHER MIND–BODY MEDICINES FOR PANIC

In addition to 5-HTP, passion flower, lemon balm, rhodiola, and ashwagandha, you may want to consider also going to a psychopharmacologist if your panic gets out of control, for temporary medication support. But warning—try to avoid Xanax, Valium, Klonopin, and other benzodiazepines. Yes, they may help in the short term, but if you find that you're using them for a very long term to curb anxiety and panic, you may find out, as I've said, that you end up getting two problems instead of one. In addition to PTSD, you might find out you have an addiction, and then you'll end up having to go to rehab to get off the Xanax, Valium, or Klonopin. Not easy.

Traditional Chinese medicine can be helpful to treat brain and body anxiety, especially after panic. Try these:

- If you tend to get hot/cold sweats—zizyphi spinosae
- If you tend to get shortness of breath and panic—lumbricus
- If your blood pressure tends to be too high or you get chest symptoms—uncariae
- If you have problems falling asleep—magnetium
- If you have stomach distress and panic—os draconis and concha ostrea

If you're perimenopausal, and you have symptoms of anxiety and panic from PTSD, there are a variety of other medicines. Corydalis tuber treats nervousness, agitation, insomnia, and headache. Coptidis rhizome treats nervousness, anxiety, chest pressure, hot flashes, and memory issues. Then magnolia cortex promotes relaxation, decreases anxiety, and helps with insomnia as well as the stomach upset.

The Affirmations

When it comes to handling trauma, the first thing Louise does is have a person re-create it in herself and in her world. To help a person handle trauma from the past, especially childhood, she helps them create a "healthier inner child," one with memories of safety and security. Other therapies do the same. They call it "re-parenting yourself." Louise's affirmations for the inner child help you establish thought patterns in your brain for the child in you who saw the world as anxious and fearful. So, before we get to those exercises, is there really a way that that could affect your brain? Is there really a way that healing the inner child with affirmations could really rewire the injured brain circuitry of a person who has PTSD? Quite possibly, yes. There is a lot of science to suggest that past trauma changes the way we perceive the world. When you have trauma at a young age, the memory warps your brain circuits. Affirmations help you change the wiring.

So perhaps by doing these inner child exercises, we are implanting in our brain competing thoughts and memories that dilute or drown out traumatic ones. I don't think you can ever remove a traumatic memory. Many wonderful, brilliant, and great people's lives have been formed and directed by trauma. Nelson Mandela, for one, was imprisoned for 25 years and, to say the least, was subjected to catastrophic humiliation and physical and emotional suffering that later took its toll on his physical health. And his trauma gave birth to a form of wisdom that is a revolutionary force to create peace in our society. You don't want to remove all your traumatic memory, do you? If you do, think again. Erasing traumatic memory may remove sources of wisdom that could inform your future avocation or calling. Once again, try a dialectic: I personally can certainly understand the desire to wipe out pain and suffering in one's past—*and* (notice I didn't say "but") I choose instead to think of all the sundry painful and traumatic events in my life as, in fact, a credential. Many people think my best credentials are my B.A. from Brown University, my M.D. or my Ph.D. and certification in psychiatry. That may be true, *and* you may also agree that I've received wisdom in some other critical ways:

- Scoliosis and having a rod in my spine with a fusion from my neck all the way through

- Epilepsy and narcolepsy, where I "fall asleep," once falling asleep while running across a bridge and getting hit by a truck and thrown 86 feet, fracturing my pelvis, ribs, and scapula and probably sustaining a brain injury

- Bilateral invasive breast cancer with a double mastectomy and reconstruction

- During one spinal fusion revision surgery, bleeding out on the table, taking 10 minutes to be resuscitated, and being in the ICU for two and a half weeks

- Foot-long clot in a vein in my left hip

- Four small bowel obstructions

- Dyslexia and ADHD

Suffice it to say, it's been a bit of a ride. I managed to survive, maybe even thrive, despite the fact that I have a lot of scars on my body and my brain, and yes, maybe a vulnerability in my spirit, though I wouldn't want to admit it. I bring to you this credential. Now join me in Louise's meditation.

In the exercise below, Louise tries to help us rewire our brains' vision, hearing, and memory circuits by guiding us through an inner child meditation; she tries to re-create a safer and more loving world. Perhaps she is helping us rewire our amygdala and hippocampus circuits as we "re-parent" ourselves.

See your inner child. Notice how the little child looks and feels. Comfort your child. You might apologize to your little one for having neglected it for so long and only berated it and scolded it in the past. But now you can promise your inner child that from now on, you will always be there for it, you will never leave it alone, and whenever this child wants your comfort or advice or playtime with you, you will always be there. You acknowledge that this relationship with your inner child is one of the most important in your life. Tell your child how much you treasure it. Build its self-esteem and self-worth with praise. See your child relaxed, safe, peaceful, enjoying itself, laughing, happy, playing with friends, and running free. Enjoying everything it does, school, studying, being creative, sharing with others, touching a flower, hugging a tree, picking a piece of fruit, eating with delight, playing with a puppy or a kitten, or swinging a swing high above, laughing with joy, running up to you, giving you a big hug. See the two of you, healthy, living in a beautiful, safe place, having wonderful relationships, parents, friends, co-workers, being greeted with joy wherever you go. Having a special kind of love with a special person.

Now visualize the teenager within you, being comforted as it moves through the bewildering time of puberty that marks the transition from childhood to adulthood, building its self-esteem and self-worth. Visualize the adult in you now with love and congratulate yourself for having come this far. You were always doing the best you could at any point in time and space. Build your own self-esteem and self-worth. The love and acceptance you have for yourself now will make it easy to move in the next level of self-love. You are very powerful. You have the power within you to help create the kind of world you want all of us to live in.

Louise also offers affirmations for PTSD:

I am harmless to others and others are harmless to me. I feel safe with the young and with the old. I feel safe with those who are like me and those who are different from me. I feel safe with animals, I feel relaxed with animals, I live in harmony with all animals. The weather is my friend. I am in harmony with all of life—the sun, the moon, the winds and the rain and the earth and the movement of the earth. I am at peace with the elements. I am always comfortable in any weather. My body adjusts to the outer temperature. I am at ease.

I have also learned to be tranquil. In the midst of chaos, I can be tranquil. Tranquility is inner peace. I practice being peaceful when others are agitated. I do not have to buy into people's agitation. For me, peace of mind and loving myself is the most important state I can experience. By changing my thoughts, I now create peace in my world. Peace replaces fear, terror is replaced by tranquility, scariness becomes serenity, uncertainty becomes confidence. Love replaces hate. Repression makes for freedom. I bless all people with love, I surround the planet with love. I know we are safe. All is well, and so it is.

IV. Panic after a Life-Threatening Illness

Serious illness is a reasonable cause of panic, and (as you'll realize in Chapter 6) serious illness in your body may elicit anxiety in your biochemistry even if you are confident that you'll survive and maintain your physical integrity. See if the following statements apply to you.

Mind Symptoms

- You have, or you have had, an illness that has threatened your life or stopped you in your tracks.

- The health problem makes you feel alone and in the dark as to what your future may bring.

- You've been hurt by the treatment, and/or you're afraid of future treatments.

- You're afraid of what the doctors are going to tell you, and you avoid practitioners because you don't want any more bad news.

BODY SYMPTOMS

- Any of the physical symptoms of anxiety you read about in the previous sections.

If this applies to a loved one rather than to you, the panic is in essence the same, because empathically, if a loved one has a life-threatening illness, you may carry the worry and terror for him or her. Here's just a brief list of life-threatening illnesses that may affect you or your loved one:

- A diagnosis of autoimmune disease that can progress to organ failure; life-threatening allergies that prevent you from being in public

- Infertility, the loss of reproductive function

- A sexually transmitted disease whose shame is so horrifying that it prevents you from wanting to engage in intimate relationships

- Severe reflux that can progress to a variety of life-threatening stomach problems; diarrhea, constipation, or other digestive problems that prevent you from being around people

- Obesity with weight in excess of 100 pounds over your normal weight

- Heart attack, blocked coronary arteries, repeated strokes

- Cancers of any kind

- Progressive memory loss, Parkinson's disease, dementias

If this is the situation you are in (or a loved one is in) and you're having trouble managing your anxiety and terror, to the point that it's making it hard for you to handle your life in the face of a complicated health problem, read on. (And just a hint: your anxiety is not all in your head.)

EVAN: I'M AFRAID I'M GOING TO DIE

Evan called my medical intuitive service, panicking, wanting a reading right away.

THE INTUITIVE READING

When I looked at Evan emotionally, all I could see was fear and dread, fear and dread. I had a hard time seeing his life. I knew that he was looking at his mortality, which was rare for him. I saw that he was a person who was very, very driven, someone who was fiercely competitive in nature, very good in a dog-eat-dog world, but not as good at seeing the spiritual and emotional side of life.

THE BODY

I sensed that Evan had trouble with focus and attention, but that could be his intense anxiety. My attention was drawn directly to his lungs, which seemed to be "dark." Was this because he lived in a smoky place? Did he used to smoke? The rest of his body didn't seem to be an issue.

THE FACTS

Evan said, "I'm afraid I'm going to die." Evan told me he had been diagnosed with a shadow on his lung after years of smoking. A biopsy revealed he had lung cancer. He was getting ready to see an oncologist. Evan was a very successful businessman who had bought and sold real estate for years. He said he had spent all of his life working, working, working, and really never got to know his children or his partner. Now that he was alone, divorced, and his children had grown up, he was afraid that he might die alone. His entire life, he'd always felt like he was in control—in control of the business deal, able to maintain a stoic face in the midst of fierce competition—but now, faced with a life-threatening illness and potential mortality, he felt terrified of losing control and very alone.

EXISTENTIAL FEAR

Are you stopped in your tracks by panic in the face of a life-threatening illness? At some time in all of our lives, we're going to have the fear of bodily harm, the fear of our mortality, the fear of a loved one's death, the fear of our own death. All of us come to this planet, we are born, but then one day, of course, we have to leave the planet; we have to die. Evan's story reminds me of that David Bowie song "The Man Who Sold the World." I had to play this song nine times before I got any idea of what it might mean. The song is about someone who never loses control. It's about a man who creates an identity he shows to the world. But that identity is one-dimensional, because it's only about "I," what he does for work, what he does when he comes home. It's never about "we." It's not two-dimensional, or it's not about we, him in spirit. So, in fact, he sold out. He sold his identity to be a lawyer, to be wealthy, rather than to be in a relationship with somebody else or with spirit. The man who sold the world.

Are you facing fear of an illness? That proverbial crossroads in life? You may be asking yourself, *Is this all there is? How much more time do I have left? What do I want to do with it?*

THE SOLUTION

Fear of death is not a psychiatric problem. However, if you are suffering from a life-threatening illness, your brain-body chemistry may be disrupted to such a degree that you may have problems with anxiety, not to mention brain fog. Ironically, in the midst of the crisis in your health, it may be hard to know where panic and terror end and health problems begin. You may not even know you have brain fog that is making it hard for you to emotionally, mentally, and spiritually see your way through this developmental stage in your life, one all of us sooner or later have to face.

Don't go it alone. Have a health team where you are the CEO. Mind you, you will call the shots and they will be advisors. Have one of the physicians or practitioners evaluate you for delirium or brain fog. If that's you, go to the previous case in this chapter and follow the suggestions in that section. Make sure you get continuous support so people can help you focus and keep track of details as you progress through your healing journey.

DEPRESSION AND ANXIETY

As you make adjustments to family, relationships, finances, and career, it's normal to get depressed and anxious. But anxiety and depression can be a sign that your body's chemistry is out of balance. (See Chapter 1.) Have a counselor you feel comfortable with support you through the grief and panic that's inevitable during this journey. Resist the need to overmedicate with supplements, herbs, or medicines during this time, as these substances may over-cloud your mind. However, consider taking some small amount of the anxiety solutions in the first case in this chapter.

Get social support. A friend or buddy can help reduce anxiety and improve longevity.[5] The absence of close friends affects our longevity as much as alcohol, obesity, or cigarette smoking. This is when a close friend holding your hand will do as much for your anxiety as for extending your life.

Get a spiritual advisor. When the friends have left and you're home or in a room alone, you may feel particular terror and anxiety. No matter who or what you believe in, a health crisis challenges anybody's faith. Even the most devoutly spiritual individuals may lose their faith or at least question it during a health crisis. Alternately, someone who previously had no faith at all—a devout atheist, you might say—may start to question whether there's more. This may be the moment in which you need an advisor to bat back and forth these ideas. Yes, it's great to bat them around in a journal, alone, but the healing power of sitting with another person may help clear your way toward finding some peace in what may feel at times like an abyss. Christian mystics called life crisis such as a life-threatening illness the "dark night of the soul." Find illumination and solace, be it from a spiritual advisor, a pastor, or simply a friend.

Did I Cause My Illness?

In medical intuition, a life-threatening illness has to do with getting in touch with your purpose in life, why you are here, but also getting in touch with your higher power, God, whatever you want to call it. The very fact of fearing death makes a person feel powerless. In the 12-step tradition, whether it's dealing with alcoholism or any other addiction, the first step is realizing your life is unmanageable, out of control, and you understand that there is a power greater than you. Some people have difficulty understanding this concept, so they try to find how or why they caused their problem. It's not either-or. If it's difficult for you, understand that we co-create our life in partnership with a greater source, a higher power. You have some influence on your life, but a higher power, the whole universe, also adds its influence, and together you create in partnership. Would you agree that you don't have an equal vote with the whole universe? I don't know—I don't have all the answers, because I'm not dead yet! I'm still trying to find them as I grow and gain more wisdom through these "learning experiences" in life. If you too are facing a life-threatening illness, understand that none of us have all the answers. Affirmations help calm us just a little bit, give us solace, as we face a life-threatening illness and handle a potential transition in our life. Affirmations do not prevent us from dying from a life-threatening illness. Prayer does not prevent us from dying. Affirmations, like prayer, help us develop our full mind-body potential during life-threatening illness, which is in a way a developmental stage of our life.

The Affirmations

Louise offers these affirmations for a life-threatening illness:

I feel safe in my body. I am healthy and safe and secure. Old beliefs, and disease, and pain, and suffering are now released. I now choose to be healthy and I now radiate vibrant health. I take loving care of my body and my body loves me. Food is my friend. Exercise is my friend. I am safe when exercising. I enjoy the feeling of exercise. My body loves to be stretched and

I choose exercise that is a joy. It is safe for me to be young. It is safe for me to be old. I look forward to living a long and healthy life. Every age holds its own joys and treasures. I will enjoy my life to its last minute and beyond, and when I leave this world, I know I will be safe in my next new adventure. When it is time to make my transition, I will pass from this world in peace and in harmony at that time that is perfect for me. Death is a natural experience and I am safe. Life gives me all of my experiences at the perfect time. I am in harmony with this process called life, and even though sometimes I do not understand why certain things happen, I am willing to see beyond it and know that life is always unfolding at my highest good. I no longer choose to scare myself with my own thoughts. I love myself too much to frighten myself ever again. I see myself standing in a very safe place, releasing burdens and pain and fear. Old negative addictions and patterns, seeing them falling away from me, and then seeing myself standing there with my arms wide open, saying I am open and receptive too, and declaring for myself what it is I want, not what I don't want, but what I do want, and know that it is possible. I see myself whole and healthy at peace. I see myself filled with love. I see a connection with other people and feel the love that is in this world and I know that I'm part of it, and the love that is in this world can move from heart to heart, and as my love goes around this world, it comes back to me multiplied in an incredible circle of love. I see myself in the center of this circle, surrounded by love, safe, at peace, and in harmony with all of life. I have the ability to love my life and to love myself. And so it is.

$$\boxed{\textit{Chapter 3}}$$

ADDICTION

Do any of these behaviors sound familiar to you? Is there anything on this list that you focus on to the exclusion of what could make you happy in your life, whether it's family, friends, or a productive career?

- Collecting shoes, clothes, books, technology (yet another new device), sports activities (like hiking or running), maybe even self-inflicted injuries

- Texting, social media, checking e-mail, shopping, sex, pornography

- Dieting, bulimia, alcohol, illicit drugs, coffee and colas, carbohydrates, chocolate, smoking, working, betting, gambling

- Rescuing people, needing to be needed, not wanting to be alone

- Gossiping, talking on the phone

- Lying, stealing, shoplifting, speeding, smartphone apps, video games, Internet surfing, risky behavior

- Perpetual spiritual practices that facilitate your avoiding or escaping life on earth

Now, when it comes to the thing on this list that you fear you might have a problem with, ask yourself the following questions:

- Have you ever felt the need to Cut down on doing it?

- Have people Annoyed you by criticizing you for it?

- Have you ever felt Guilty about it?

- When you wake up in the morning, is the first thing you think about when you open your Eyes?

You just gave yourself the CAGE questionnaire. CAGE is usually used to identify alcohol addiction; however, though the questionnaire is not valid for diagnosing other addictions, modified versions of it have been used to identify other addictions in one form or another. If you say yes to two or more of those questions, it indicates you may have a problem. And the most important question in the CAGE questionnaire is number 4—the eye-opener. Because if what's consuming you is the first thing you think about when you open your eyes in the morning—*hello*?

If one of these behaviors has hijacked your life and taken over your time, money, resources, so that it's hard for you to have a full life with family, friends, money, work, and so on, chances are addiction to some degree has affected you. If you have trouble breaking the cycle of eating, drinking, or doing any of the things I just listed, then join the club. Is there any one of us who doesn't have an addiction or two?

WAYS OF LOOKING AT ADDICTION

Addictions are a key part of our intuitive guidance system letting us know we are covering up a feeling that we can't handle. Addiction is an attempt to use something, anything, to cover up a feeling—maybe even emptiness—inside you. Ask yourself, is it food that's filling up the emptiness? Is it alcohol? Is it gambling?

Is it drugs? Or maybe it's that relationship that is bad for you. Or do you always have to rescue people in need? Or is it the continual buying of things, saving and collecting and storing things in your house? Whatever it is, we all have to come to grips with those elements in our lives that have gotten out of control like weeds in the garden: drinking, eating, relating, whatever it is that is addictively filling up the emotional and spiritual emptiness.

We often use drinking, eating, sex, pills, gambling, excessive working, excessive anything to give us a love reward that we don't have inside us. The brain chemistry for addiction is the same for love and reward, for self-nurturance, and the connection with the divine. According to Louise Hay, addictive behavior is another way of saying, "I'm not good enough." When you get caught up in this kind of behavior, what you're really trying to do is run away from your feelings. Think about it the next time you eat too much popcorn or troll Facebook for too many hours yet again, or spend too much money on shoes or clothing you don't need, or whatever your addiction is. What are you escaping?

At first your go-to addiction is very rewarding. It really hits the spot. Whether it is that first cigarette, that first drink, the first time you had sex with that person, the first time you pulled that lever in the slot machine, you felt that thrill. Then, of course, you find yourself doing more and more of the behavior and feeling less and less of the thrill. That's because the hallmark of addiction is you build up tolerance. The same amount of drinking, sex, buying, or eating gives you less and less relief over time, so you have to use more and more to get the same effect. But what's worse is you can't stop. If you stop drinking, buying, eating, or having sex with that person, you feel awful. You go through a kind of emotional and physical withdrawal, with painful symptoms of emotional and physical distress.

We usually think that addiction or abuse is just a psychological problem. No. Addiction rewires our brains, whether it's alcohol, cocaine, gambling, or sex, unwanted changes occur in our brain and our body, our psyche and our spirit. Circuits in your brain that function for relationships, work, learning, and so on—those brain pathways get taken up by acquiring your go-to substance. Literally, your brain gets hijacked by your addiction. So instead of you getting love and fulfillment through family, relationships, work, and so on, your time and your brain chemistry gets taken up by your substance, whether it's alcohol, sex, gambling, whatever. But there's a solution. You can rewire your brain in a healthier way, away from compulsive desire for something that in the end makes you a slave to it.

REASONS FOR ADDICTION

Why do we have addictions in the first place? Every one of us has some unique difference about our brain that makes it hard for us to adapt. Some people have social anxiety. With an imbalance in the GABA receptor, they may use alcohol, which hits the GABA receptor to ease their embarrassment in social situations. Similarly, people with attention deficit disorder (we haven't gotten to that chapter yet) may have disorders of dopamine, another neurotransmitter, so they may try to jerry-rig their brain into working by using substances that balance their neurochemistry, whether it's nicotine, caffeine, cocaine, or amphetamines. Individuals with ADHD shop around for a drug that will sharpen their minds. Last but not least, people with depression might have problems with serotonin. And, of course, eating carbohydrates—pasta, rice, bread, or sweets—may make our bodies boost serotonin levels and lift our moods, as well as boost our waistlines.

So is that it? Do you have to have anxiety, depression, or ADHD to have an addiction? Of course not. You don't have to have a diagnosis to misuse a substance to cover up some emotion that you're uncomfortable with. All of us have some emotion or other that we're uncomfortable with. So we troll the face of the earth to find something that helps us bide our time, makes it easier to be human. Addictions have been around since probably the cavemen and cavewomen. Probably cave dogs and cave cats as well. Have you noticed that when your dog or cat gets depressed, he hits the kibble more? Your brain pathways are some of the most primitive (pun intended) areas of your brain involving opiates and dopamine. Opiates and dopamine involve the most basic areas for survival: love, nurturance, relationships, and reward. If these needs aren't met, we simply don't feel alive.

We might succumb to alcohol or drugs because our friends are using them. That's what they call the peer pressure part of addiction. Or we might find that we turn to alcohol, pills, or sex because we are in perpetual pain. Many people who have had minor surgery and have used oxycodone or Percocet find that they stay hooked on the drugs because they also remove the emotional pain of being in a bad relationship. Others are just bored with their lives, and the numbing, nonstimulating pain of boredom is easily replaced by the escapism of hallucinogens and other stimulating substances. Some people want to use substances to connect to the divine, with peyote or other psychedelic substances. People since the beginning of time have used substances to seek a spiritual experience. Some people addictively involve themselves in spirituality in such a way that it supplants involvement in relationships, a productive vocation, and relationships on planet Earth in general. Ironically, the great psychiatrist and substance abuse expert Abraham Twerski, a rabbi, said that our craving for the divine is the basis for addiction—that when we have a sense of emptiness in our lives, and boredom, we really don't know that emptiness is a lack of connection to spirit. To fill that inner craving we can't name, many people turn to drugs. He called this the spiritual anatomy of addiction.

ADDICTION AND MEDICAL INTUITION

According to medical intuition, addiction is a key part of our intuitive guidance system that lets us know we're having a hard time balancing our self, our self-love, with our ability to handle work or responsibility to others. It's a third-center issue. As you remember from the introduction, the health of the third center involves balancing our self-esteem or self-love with our ability to feel responsibility for others. If we have difficulty handling that balance, we're more like to suffer from problems with weight, digestion, and body image, but also addiction. Whether it's diabetes, which is a pancreas problem, or the effects of alcohol on the liver, the stomach, or the pancreas, all things addiction are third center.

In the brain, addiction involves opiates from the nucleus accumbens and dopamine from the ventral tegmentum. But reward doesn't just come from brain neurochemistry. We can feel reward from children, pets, work, activism in the world, a relationship, family, learning, spirituality, nature—every emotional center in medical intuition has a source for reward. Mind-body health involves having happiness, a rewarding life, via multiple areas of our life. Like having a balanced stock portfolio, we have to have multiple areas that we invest ourselves in emotionally. If you find yourself only getting reward from one area, that is, work *or* sex *or* helping people, you are in essence getting reward from only one center. Since there are seven centers in medical intuition, each one contributes 14 percent of our life. If all of your focus, for example, is on your relationship (second center; 14 percent), and it's hijacking your energy so you have no other emotional, physical, or financial resources for the other centers, (1, 3, 4, 5, 6, 7; 86 percent), some label this a relationship addiction. Yes, you can have an artificial sense of reward or opiates when we do cocaine, gamble, have sex, or rescue others. However, you're not fooling yourself. If you don't have happiness and reward in multiple balanced, healthy areas of your life, you'll soon suffer from addiction.[1]

THE ANATOMY OF LOVE AND ADDICTION

Louise Hay says addiction is inner emptiness and damaged self-love. What is self-love, anyway? You know what Tina Turner says in "What's Love Got to Do with It?" Is love a secondhand emotion? No, it's a firsthand emotion. When you're born, you look at your mother, your mother looks at you, and you start to develop self-love right then and there. The biology of self-love begins with opiates. Yes, it's that same neurotransmitter for addiction. Right away, from the very moment you're born, when you look at someone else and they look at you, the wiring for self-love begins to course through your brain and body. Then, when you develop language, all the words that you use for how you feel about yourself and others start to wire self-love or self-esteem in your brain and body. If you say, "I hate myself. I hate my hips. I hate my abdomen. I'm stupid. I'm dumb," your sense of self-love plummets and so do your internalized opiates and dopamine. You may then try to import your neurochemistry of self-love artificially through food, through drugs, or through other addictions. This is the anatomy of trying to fake yourself into believing you love yourself, but it's not lasting. The drugs soon wear off. When that relationship leaves you, and you're alone, you then have to face yourself, and that deep emptiness inside you exposes your lack of self-love.

The antithesis of self-love is shame. Shame is believing that you have something defective about you. Guilt, humiliation, whatever it is, you think something is wrong about you. *I feel shame about my hips, I feel shame about my intellect. I feel shame about some aspect of my history that I feel is awful, is abhorrent.* And then you start to believe that other people think there's something wrong with you too. They're laughing at you. They're criticizing you. They're judging you. All of this becomes wired in your brain and body. Low self-esteem, shame, criticism, blah, blah, blah. And then you end up trying to medicate this ball of bad emotions with addiction. Ultimately, a lack of self-love breeds low self-esteem, which breeds addiction.[2]

So, you may be able to take a fearless inventory of why you have a problem with addiction, whether it's food, drink, alcohol, drugs, gambling, sex, cigarettes, bad relationships, and so on. But, ultimately, knowing why you have an addiction doesn't give you the skills to get rid of it. Knowing you're genetically prone to addiction, knowing that you had a traumatic past, knowing that you have a history of depression, anxiety, or ADHD doesn't give you the skills to manage your addiction any more than knowing why you got that flat tire helps you fix the tire. Change the tire now and then figure out where the nail came from. Manage your addiction now so it can give you the skills and the emotional resilience to be able to handle your past, if you even want to. Yes, it's true. If you look at the origins of the addiction, it can help to buffer your brain into place while you're getting addiction treatment.

Some addiction is called "dual diagnosis." That's right, two diagnoses, not one. For people who have anxiety and addiction, their dual diagnosis would mean that they are more likely to have alcohol addiction because alcohol hits the GABA receptor, influencing anxiety. Similarly, someone who has problems with sex addiction would be more likely to have problems with opiates. Finally, someone who has problems with overeating, especially "comfort food," is probably more likely to have a history of trauma and depression. What do I mean by comfort food? In the event that you don't know what comfort food is, look it up on the web. In any case, often comfort foods are used addictively. They are the cornerstone of our current epidemic of obesity. Sixty percent of the United States has a problem with obesity, and it's not because of a lack of information. Often it's because food is being used to fill up that emptiness in self-esteem and disappointment about ourselves and about love we get from others. Look at what you're drawn to, addictively, the neurochemistry of it. Is it alcohol? Then chances are you're medicating anxiety. Is it potatoes, pasta, rice, Cinnabon? Then chances are you are medicating something else: sadness, shame, lost love? Irritability, distractibility, brain fog? The anatomy of craving tells you what the other side of your dual diagnosis is, what chemistry in your brain you're trying to solve.

ADDICTIONS AND AFFIRMATIONS

There are many kinds of addictions beside chemical ones. There are pattern addictions that we adopt to keep us from being present in our lives, says Louise Hay. Business, distraction, work addiction, rescue addiction. By engaging in all of this business, this ch-ch-chatter in our brain, we can crowd out that inner voice of spiritual and intuitive wisdom. Mindfulness helps us sit in silence, stop the chatter, and listen to that single voice of the divine or our soul. If you simply can't sit in silence, if you have to crowd your life with this chitter-chatter, chitter-chatter, chitter-chatter of business, rescuing, loud noises, then you are using pattern addictions to escape emotions you can't handle.

Louise Hay has some positive affirmations for addiction. These include:

- We are each responsible for our experiences.

- Every thought we think is creating our future.

- Everyone is dealing with the damaging patterns of resentment, criticism, guilt, and self-hatred.

- These are only thoughts, and thoughts have been changed.

- We need to release the past and forgive everyone, including ourselves.

- Self-approval and self-acceptance in the now are the keys to positive changes.

- The point of power is always in the present moment.

And then she says, finally, if you're going to be addicted to anything, why not be addicted to yourself? After all, loving yourself will give you the chemistry of what you are craving anyway.

TREATING ADDICTIONS

Traditionally, the first step in treating addiction is to restore, maybe even recover, a balanced brain neurochemistry and simultaneously suppress your urge to use a substance or do an unhealthy behavior. Many people think addiction is just getting you to stop drinking or doing drugs. However, that's not true. In medical intuition, addiction treatment is about third-center rehab. It's rehabilitating your self-esteem, your self-love, but also your capacity to be responsible in the world—to uphold your responsibilities, not just to yourself but to other people, your relationships, your family, your work, your bills, and so on.

There are several prototypical treatments. The most common is the 12-step program. In a 12-step group, people recognize that their lives have become unmanageable, and in a partnership with a higher power, they submit to a series of cognitive and spiritual improvements. What does that mean? You rewire your brain and you get in contact with spirit or a power greater than you. Many people have trouble with this concept. Well, a famous story that's been bandied around 12-step programs is this: A man stood up and said, "I don't know. I have trouble with the whole God/spiritual power thing." So a woman stands up and says, "Would you agree that you ain't him?" The point is, you can probably agree that somewhere out there there's a power greater than you.

Another source of help for addiction is psychiatry, a dual diagnosis program. So, if you have depression and addiction, or anxiety and addiction, anger, ADHD—the list is very long—a psychiatrist or other licensed practitioner will help you pharmacologically treat that disorder, targeting GABA, dopamine, serotonin, and other medicines and nutritional supplements. However, a reputable practitioner will only use nutritional supplements and medicines that are nonaddictive. If you find yourself trying to go to another doctor and get another medicine because that pill won't give you the same buzz as your cocaine, that drug won't give you the same euphoria as the oxycodone, et cetera, guess again. You are engaging in addictive behavior *again*. Most addiction treatment uses cognitive behavioral therapy and now dialectical behavioral therapy, in addition to affirmations, to change those thought patterns in your frontal lobe that take you away from self-love and into unbalanced ways of thinking and behaving. A technical term for this is *relapse prevention*.[3]

Last but not least, work and vocation are extremely important. If you don't have work, you will have a lot of time on your hands, and you will get those cravings. In fact, work is the most

potent "medicine" or "drug" for addiction. Why? Because rewarding work helps release opiates, that key neurochemical of addiction. You might say, "Well, I hate my work, so therefore, I won't
work." Er . . . wrong! What you need is a structured job that helps
you get up and out the door. By having a stable schedule, you'll
help reconstruct your biorhythms, those schedules for cortisol in
your brain, and rehabilitate the pathways that have been hijacked
by addiction. And while you're engaged in that job, you can work
with a vocational counselor who can help you get the right education and training to start to approach an avocation or calling
that's more in keeping with your dream career. And if work is your
addiction, your vocational counselor will help you learn to engage
with it in a healthy way.

The best thing about working in a community, a support
group, that helps with addiction is that it gives you, in fact, a
family. Most addictions run in a family, and most people experience trauma as a result of being raised in a family of addiction.
By being involved in a 12-step group, we get to have a "prosthetic family," another family that helps rehabilitate our way of
relating, out from under the influence of a substance. Many people who have addiction have fallings-out with their families of
origin, lose their spouses, and become alienated from children.
Learning how to make up for that injury that has happened in a
relationship and build new bonds is essential for the treatment
of addiction.

THE MEDICINES

There are a variety of medicines used for a person staying in
remission. Whether it's Suboxone, methadone, naloxone, and so
on, all of these medicines bind to the opiate receptor and report-
edly make a person less likely to relapse. However, medicines
alone are not going to change your behavior. It's well known
that many people use any and all of these medicines and then
still use the substance of abuse. The cornerstone of addiction is

rehabilitating a person's third center: his or her self-love, self-image, responsibility to others, as well as to vocation, relationships, and family.

Rome was not built in a weekend. Addiction recovery doesn't happen that way, either. The truth is, no matter what kind of assistance you are receiving, most people fall in and out of treatment. Addiction, like any illness, has many stages. I'm not going to go through all the stages. Suffice it to say that any life-threatening illness, even cancer, has various stages where a person goes in and out of remission. And addiction is a serious illness. People die from it, and the havoc it creates in the lives of the loved ones around the person with addiction is devastating. The treatment can be extremely expensive, can be very effective, and yet can take several rounds before it "takes." Don't be discouraged. There is support out there.[4]

EXERCISES FOR CHANGE

In addition to the affirmations you read above, Louise offers some powerful tools to treat addiction. The first is an exercise called "Release Your Addictions":

> This is when the changes take place, here and now in your own mind. Take some deep breaths, close your eyes, and think about the person, place, or thing you're addicted to. Think of the insanity behind the addiction. You are trying to fix what you think is wrong inside of you by grabbing on to something that is outside of you. The point of power is in the present moment, and you can begin to make a shift today. Once again, by being willing to release the need, say, "I am willing to release the need for X (that's your addiction) in my life. I release it now and trust in the process of light to meet my needs." Say it every morning in your daily affirmations and prayers. You have taken another step to freedom.

Another exercise that can help you forgive and release is "Your Secret Addiction":

List 10 secrets that you have never shared with anyone regarding your addiction. If you are an overeater, maybe you have eaten out of a garbage can. If you are an alcoholic, you may have kept alcohol in the car so you could drink while driving. If you are a compulsive gambler, perhaps you put your family into jeopardy in order to borrow money to continue your addiction. List 10 secrets. How do you feel now? Look at your worst secret. Visualize yourself in this period of your life and love that person. Tell them how much you love and forgive. Look into the mirror and say, "I forgive you and love you exactly as you are. Breathe."

Many people have told Louise they can't enjoy today because of something that happened in the past. But holding on to the past only hurts us. It means we're refusing to live in the moment. The past is over and cannot be redone. You can start releasing the past with an exercise called "Ask Your Family":

Let's go back to your childhood for a moment and ask a few questions. Fill in the blanks:

1. My mother always made me _____.

2. What I really wanted her to say was _____.

3. What she really didn't know was _____.

4. My father told me I shouldn't _____.

5. If my father only knew _____.

6. I wish I could have told my father _____.

7. Mother, I forgive you for _____.

8. Father, I forgive you for _____.

9. What would you still like to tell your parents about yourself? What is the unfinished business that you still have?

These exercises help you address your addiction and also help you address your self-esteem. In medical intuition, as we've seen, self-esteem and addiction are in the same center. By rewiring your self-esteem, you are mirroring the neurochemistry that you've been importing through your addiction. Try this exercise, "Self-Approval/Self-Esteem Rehabilitation":

> Every time you think about your addiction for the next month, say over and over to yourself, "I approve of myself." Say this 300 or 400 times a day. No, it's not too many times. When you are worrying, you will go over your problem at least that many times in a day. Let "I approve of myself" become a walking mantra, something that you say over and over to yourself almost nonstop. Saying "I approve of myself" is guaranteed to bring up everything in your consciousness that is in opposition. When a negative thought like "How can you approve of yourself? You spent all that money." Or "You just ate two pieces of cake!" or "You'll never amount to anything!" or whatever your negative battle may be, this is the time to take mental control. Give it no importance. Just say the thought for what it is, another way to keep you stuck in the past. Gently say to this thought, "Thank you for sharing. I let you go. I approve of myself." These thoughts of resistance will have no power over you unless you choose to believe them.

THE ALL IS WELL CLINIC

I. THE EATING ADDICTIONS

There are so many disorders of eating. Whether it's simply binge eating versus anorexia, bulimia, compulsive eating, addictive eating, or simply out-of-control, imbalanced, obsessive-compulsive nutritional and dietary practices, it can be a product of trying to medicate one's depression (Chapter 1), anxiety (Chapter 2), attention problems (Chapter 4), or, in the case of this chapter, addiction. I've found in my 30-plus years working as a medical intuitive and in psychiatry that I find myself saying, more frequently than not, almost all roads end in addiction. Meaning that all of us have some form of addiction. In this section we discuss eating first, because all of us have to do it—that is, eat. And therefore food is probably the most common abused and misused substance that we have to cover up an emotion we can't handle. We all need food with which to exist. And as with work or relationships, we also need food to survive, thrive, and be healthy.

Learning how to handle eating and drinking for satiety and sobriety is not always an issue. Some of us, genetically or by a quirk of fate, are able to get through life without having some form of disordered eating. However, given that 60 percent of at least the United States, with the world rapidly catching up, is overweight, near obese, it's clear that the addiction of disordered eating has wide ramifications to affect our health and longevity.

Do the following statements apply to you?

MIND SYMPTOMS

- You're embarrassed about how much you eat or what you eat, so much that often you'll only eat certain foods alone.

- Often after eating you're disgusted with yourself, depressed, or feeling guilty.

- At times, you can find yourself eating an amount of food that's obviously larger than what most people eat during that time.

- Often when you eat, you lack control and you can't stop.

- Go back to the beginning of the chapter and ask yourself the CAGE questions when it comes to your eating. Have you tried to Cut back? Have you felt Annoyed? Guilty about what and how much you eat? Thinking about it first thing when you open your Eyes? Then chances are food is an obsession for you, your behavior around it is a compulsion, and your addictive use of it is eventually going to affect your health.

BODY SYMPTOMS

- Physically you can't stop eating until you feel uncomfortably full.

- Physically you eat large amounts of food even when you're not hungry.

- Physically you're not even aware when you are eating. You may find that before you know it, a whole bowl of popcorn or carton of ice cream is gone. You won't even remember where all those cookies went. It's as if your eating is on autopilot.

If this is you, you're not alone, and you know it. If you've ever been on a sports team or in a dorm, you're well aware of how much socialization goes on around food. And how, when people get stressed, they take breaks from their "anxiety" and immerse themselves in the bowl of popcorn, the ice cream, the chocolate-chip cookies, and so on. And then once we graduate and we leave the dorm, our groups, and our buddies behind, we go off to live alone or with our partners, and we end up doing the same behaviors, often, trying to secretly hide what we've been doing for years—that is, bingeing large amounts of food during times of anxiety or stress. Some of us do periodic cleanses to "reset" our metabolism from this excessive intake of calories, but after this "fast" of greatly reduced calories, we need to "reward" ourselves, which leads to another binge. And this is in our 20s and 30s. This cycle of stress – excessive eating – binge – shame – guilt – cleanse, this yo-yo up-and-down dieting, distorts your metabolism as much as it distorts your brain circuits for mood, reward, body image, and self-esteem. And then, by the time you hit 40 or 50 and your hormones start to change, you're left with a Bermuda Triangle of disrupted metabolism, disrupted brain circuits for eating and addiction, disrupted mood, anxiety, and attention, not to mention hormones. Read on to the following case for a problem that so many of us are oh so familiar with.

JILL: BINGE EATING

Jill, 32, called me because she was having trouble losing weight.

THE INTUITIVE READING

When I looked at Jill's life, I saw early in her life that she had been the "scapegoat" in her family. It felt like she had had a falling-out with the major person in charge, someone who felt like a king or queen. Jill felt like she was the one singled out for criticism and shame. No matter what she did, it was never good enough.

THE BODY

Jill's mind felt like a hummingbird that never rested. Her posture appeared to slump, and I sensed a lump in her throat. Her lower extremities felt like lead. I saw that she craved carbohydrates, such as pasta, rice, bread, or sweets, to soothe moodiness, irritability, and sadness. The moodiness and irritability seemed to make her adrenal gland convert body fat to estrogen and cortisol that affected her breast tissue and her hormones. I saw that she had blood sugar swings.

THE FACTS

Jill told me that she ate compulsively and had spent many years hiding food from her roommates. Struggling with her weight all of her life, she managed to lose 70 pounds and then gain it all back. Recently, her mother had rejected Jill for marrying a man because she "hated him." Her mother's exact words were "You're dead to me now." Since she married her husband, Jill had been totally ostracized by her family, and after her wedding, that's when the pounds really began to pile on, and Jill developed hormonal problems too. When she developed two breast lumps, the doctors said they were related to excess weight.

In the United States, obesity and weight problems are at the top of the list. When most people talk about their health, they rarely talk about their weight. They'll talk about knee pain, lower back pain, ankle issues, breast lumps, heavy menstrual flow, digestive symptoms, hypertension, and cholesterol, but they rarely talk about their weight when they list their health problems, and weight or excessive body fat is usually the one cause of any or all of these problems.[5]

If you have problems with weight, chances are you've tried over and over to lose it. You're embarrassed or frustrated if someone brings it up. And though you've spent years, perhaps decades, of your life feeling guilty when you do eat, you've already done everything you can to try to lose the weight or the body fat. So when it comes to thinking about your health, somehow weight doesn't come on the list because it's such a frustrating problem, you try to put it out of your mind. It's as if all the other issues in your health—breast lumps, knee pain, ankle pain, hypertension—are at least something you could do something about with medicines, nutritional supplements, or herbs. Because the solution to your weight has thus far eluded you and millions of other people, though you actually have heard of people handling and healing these other health problems. So you focus in on something that you're going to be able to solve.

And if you have problems with weight, chances are if you don't already, you will at some point have problems with chronic pain. For every 10 pounds you're overweight, it puts 40 pounds of force on your back, your knees, and your ankles. And over the years, if your weight continues to go up, your disability will increase. The leading cause of disability for people who are obese is knee osteoarthritis. Whether it's arrhythmias or cardiovascular disorders or total body inflammation, all of these disorders can be made better if we lose weight.[6] But how?

The Solution

If you are like Jill and all the rest of us, your weight problems can never be solved with just nutritional counseling. Weight is a complex brain-body disorder similar to addiction. Science has started to look at the weight-loss problem and has seen that all weight problems are not the same.[7] Some people have high insulin. Other people have difficulty responding to a sense of fullness while eating. Other individuals cannot prevent themselves from eating that tempting cupcake or French fry if they see it, while other people just follow the eating patterns of high calorie, fat, sugar, and salt that they learned as children. Some individuals (the subject of this chapter) have binge-eating disorders and food addiction. And finally, some people have difficulty with being active or find a lot of value in being sedentary. We can't lump all people with weight problems in one category. This helps explain why all treatments do not help all people lose weight.

If you have problems losing weight, it may be important for you engage with a weight-loss specialist or a bariatric center to find out which one of these categories you fall under. By getting a thorough physical examination, you can find out if you have problems with insulin, problems with feeling fullness. Working with a nutritionist, you might find out whether you have difficulty withstanding food temptations or breaking familial patterns of bad eating. Working with a counselor, a health care practitioner, and/or a dialectical behavioral therapist, you can learn the skills to balance your emotions and thoughts so they don't result in addictive behavior. Specifically, dialectical behavioral therapy can help you use mindfulness to soothe guilt, anger, and sadness, identify the thought patterns that make you feel bad about yourself, and react in the present in such a way that you don't use food compulsively to soothe emotions instead. Dialectical behavioral therapy is a class and a coach, so you'll get individual and group support in your struggle. And many eating disorder clinics use dialectical behavioral therapy as well to teach people life skills for creating healthier eating patterns.

EATING, SELF-IMAGE, AND THE BRAIN

A whole book could be written about food and the mind. I won't bore you with all those details. But I cannot underestimate the impact of eating, mood, anxiety, self-esteem, and disordered eating—their lifelong effects on the brain and body. So bear with me. If you learn how eating is wired in your brain, you will learn how to master this day-to-day function using medicine, intuition, and affirmations.

A lot of people have shame about eating, weight, and their self-image. In medical intuition, weight is a third-center issue. A lot of women always see themselves as heavy despite being a normal weight. How we see ourselves, our degree of normal weight, may parallel how lovable we sense we are. Some people believe that their sense of lovableness is proportionate to how physically attractive they see themselves as in the mirror. What you need to know is that, just like a carnival funhouse mirror, the visual areas in your brain actually distort how you look in the mirror. Now you might begin to see how the three-dimensional image you perceive of your body has to be disconnected in your brain from your sense of self-love.

Seriously. It bears repeating. Literally, it is possible for the brain areas for vision to widen your hips beyond how wide they really are, distort or distend the volume of your abdomen beyond what it really is, elongate your nose way beyond its actual length, and so on. If you've had a history of trauma, if someone has treated you in a hateful way, the brain sometimes has a peculiar way of handling that hate that came toward you. Rather than taking the negative feeling and deflecting it out of you, your brain absorbs it and combines it into your own three-dimensional perception of what you look like. So therefore, when you're a child and someone says repeatedly, "You're ugly, I hate you, you're stupid, I don't want you," your brain absorbs it like a paper towel absorbs a spill. Your brain gets saturated with that hate and you learn that you are undesirable. And that undesirability becomes reflected, like a mirror, on parts of your self: the nose, the hips, the abdomen, the pelvis, all these individual parts become a reflection of all the parts of you that you heard were unlovable. And all those statements of unlovability coalesce into that image you see in the mirror. The way you were "unloved" becomes a distorted perception of how you think your body is unlovable, and when you say to yourself in the present, "I hate my hips, I hate my abdomen, I hate my breasts," you are reenacting the past. You are hating on yourself. And your body is hearing it and absorbing it and further distorting your image in the mirror. It's like a reverse affirmation, like a negative version of Louise Hay's mirror work; you're not improving your self-esteem, you're lowering it. If this is you, if you hate or even strongly dislike your "image" however you look at it, you may turn to food to seek love and comfort.

THE BRAIN, EATING, AND EXCESS WEIGHT

Many people think being overweight is a problem that registers in your body, but it's truly a mind-body problem. If you have trouble with your weight, understand it's not just about self-image and self-esteem, it's also a biochemical mis-arrangement of dopamine, opiates, and other areas of the addiction network. Let's look at the brain areas that have to do with regulating eating. Drug companies are trying to target molecules like leptin, ghrelin, and others—molecules that regulate our sense of fullness after eating or desire to eat more. These drugs are targeted to artificially make us feel full before we really are, so we'll eat less, or to block our appetite in the first place. Most of the studies have shown, though, that drugs directed against leptin and ghrelin don't work for very long. Why? Because if you only focus on the body and weight and ignore emotions and addiction, you'll lose the battle.

That said, there are some treatments that really help when you actually have a serious weight problem. Serious obesity, when people are more than 80 to 100 pounds overweight, can shorten your lifespan by 10 or more years. Ultimately, by the time you get to that amount of weight, a more dramatic, immediate solution is needed. Ghrelin receptors are located in the stomach lining. For some people, bariatric surgery can be extremely effective because it reduces the size of the stomach, reduces the area that produces ghrelin, and may trick the brain's metabolism areas.[8]

Am I saying everyone should go out and have bariatric surgery? Hell, no! Absolutely not. What I am saying is for some people, a band procedure may be what is necessary to save their lives.

It's up to you and your physician to decide what is the next, most effective step in managing your weight long-term.[9] But whether you decide to have bariatric surgery or not, you're still going to have to address the brain-body chemistry and the self-esteem and self-image components of addiction. In the end, we all see drugs for weight loss come and go. Who hasn't heard of Fen-Phen (fenfluramine/phentermine), which was all the rage in the '80s? This drug helped people lose weight, but it also caused a life-threatening lung disease, pulmonary hypertension, so it was taken off the market. Any drug you take has its effects and its side effects, and a drug to reduce weight does as well. Which leads me to stimulants. Stimulants like Adderall and others have long been used by certain individuals to lose weight. However, after the first five pounds, people rarely lose significant amounts of weight, and then they're stuck on this medicine, which can increase the chance over time for hypertension and other heart problems.

When it comes to the brain, there are ways to reduce appetite using nutritional supplements, herbs, medicines, intuition, and affirmations. First, address the variety of food. If you want to lose weight, you're better off eating the same thing every day. I know, you're probably saying, "But that's boring." Right! You'll be bored all the way to losing a lot of weight. Diets that involve eating more or less the same food every day reduce dopamine stimulation in the reward centers, reduce your appetite, and, as a result, you lose weight. And although you say, "I don't want to eat the same food every day," it is an effective way to lose weight.[10]

Here's an effective and reasonable meal plan to rewire your brain and body toward a healthy weight. Notice I'm not using the D-word—*diet*. That word probably increases your anxiety and frustration right away, which makes your adrenal gland release cortisol, which of course increases insulin and ultimately weight. Instead, I suggest the following "meal plan," which is similar to the plan I outlined in Chapter 1. To stabilize your blood sugar and prevent you from feeling deprived:

- Eat at pretty much the same time every day.

- For breakfast, have a bowl of whole oats. If you're not allergic to dairy, drink half a glass or a full glass of low-fat milk, have a cup of coffee, and then have a bottle of water, which you drink down like a shot. Then exercise for half an hour with the tension turned all the way down on an elliptical trainer or exercise bicycle to a techno or disco beat. You can do yoga, Pilates, strength training all you want any other time during the day, but you have to do your half-hour of cardio, as they say.

- At 10 o'clock in the morning, you have a half of a protein bar. Not whole—half. And your second bottle of water, which you gulp down. You gulp the water down because it elicits a "gastrocolic reflex," which makes your colon dump digested food, thus decreasing reabsorption of fats and estrogens.

- Noon is your biggest meal of the day. No, it's not dinner. If you want to have the rest of your day to move around and not feel sluggish, lunch should be your meal of maximum volume. You take a normal dinner plate and you divide it into thirds: one-third protein, one-third carbs, one-third vegetable. If you want dessert of any kind, you take some of the carbohydrate away and have half a piece of dessert.

- At 3 o'clock in the afternoon, you have the other half of that protein bar you had at 10 and your third and final bottle of water. Mind you, this is your last carbohydrate.

- Dinner: No later than 6 P.M. It's a dessert plate: a small piece of protein, a dark leafy vegetable, but no carbohydrate. If you want to walk after dinner, you'll lose the weight.

- If you have trouble sticking to this, consider joining a support group like Curves, or Jenny Craig, or something of that nature so that the group support and the presence of other people can keep you on task. Work with someone who does cognitive behavioral therapy or dialectical behavioral therapy to teach you strategies of mindfulness to soothe anxiety, depression, or anger so you won't use food to calm yourself.

THE AFFIRMATIONS

Louise uses the following affirmations for binge eating and problems with weight:

- Obesity can have to do with fear, needing protection, running away from feelings. The affirmation for this is "I am at peace with my own feelings. I am safe where I am. I create my own security. I love and approve of myself."

- That fear may also be resistance to forgiveness. The affirmation for this is "I am protected by divine love. I am always safe and secure. I am willing to grow up and take responsibility for my life. I forgive others and I now create my own life the way I want. I am safe."

- High blood sugar reflects a longing for what might have been, a sense that no sweetness is left. The affirmation is "This moment is filled with joy. I now choose to experience the sweetness of today."

- For depression, the affirmation is "I now go beyond other people's fears and limitations. I create my own life."

- Anxiety is not trusting the flow and the process of life. The affirmation is "I love and approve of myself. I trust the process of life. I am safe."

- For attention problems, hyperactivity, feeling pressured and frantic, the affirmation is "I am safe. All pressure dissolves. I am good."

II. ADDICTION TO BEING THIN

When it comes to having a history of trauma, you don't just bring the memory of the past pain. When we experience a very painful childhood or a series of emotionally, physically, or sexually abusive relationships, we tend to, like Pac-Man, "eat" those memories and incorporate them into areas of our body. Just as in the previous section about distorted body image, hateful acts toward us can become memorialized in our eating behavior. True, we had no control in that traumatic experience in our past. But now we're going to feel more in control of our environment, especially our body, through how we handle our food.

The anxiety that comes with PTSD is soothed by a compulsive need to control the one thing that you can—that is, your body and food. You couldn't control that parent who was abusing you, you couldn't control what that painful partner was saying or doing to you, so at least you can control the grams of fat and carbohydrates you consume, not to mention the pounds or kilograms that register on the scale. And the depression that one tends to experience with trauma becomes medicated, addictively, through extreme restriction of calories. Whether it's bingeing and then purging, or anorexia, deprivation of calories induces opiates, which is the same neurochemical found in addiction. So if we have a problem with needing to be perfectly thin and then even *more* perfectly thin, we need to look at whether we are medicating a history of past trauma with obsessions and compulsions around food and elevating our mood via extremely low calorie intake and metabolism. If you think this may be you, or you're not sure, together with a friend, look at this list of emotional patterns around food.

Mind Symptoms

- You have an intense fear of gaining weight.

- You have obsessive thoughts of becoming fat, even though you are lower than the following weight calculation: you start at 100 pounds and for every inch of height over five feet you add five pounds. So for example, someone who's five feet tall would weigh on average 100 pounds, more or less. Someone who's five foot five would weigh on average 125, again, more or less. So if someone who's five foot five and 125 pounds has obsessive thoughts and worries about being fat, this may be an area of concern.

Behavior Symptoms

- You tend to go from one food plan to another, one diet to another, where you are greatly restricting your energy intake to a significantly lower and lower body weight for your age, height, and gender. You're constantly trying to Cut down on your food.

- People have been Annoyed by you constantly cutting down your food and trying to lose weight; they say you don't need to lose weight, you're already too thin.

- When you eat, even healthy fruit and vegetables and protein, you feel Guilty and feel you need to cut back.

- When you wake up in the morning, the first thing you think about when you open your Eyes is your weight and how little food you can eat that day. (Yes, this is the CAGE questionnaire.)

If this is you, then this is an area of concern. And this could apply to the majority of women, as well as more and more men, in our culture. We are daily bombarded with pictures of people in the media who are too thin, and with the latest diet to get thinner.

So if you don't have body distortion from the past, you may actually have it induced by the media in the present. Consider the following case.

KAREN: "PERFECTLY" THIN— BUT SHE DOESN'T THINK SO

Karen, 45, came to me for a reading because her mother told her to.

THE INTUITIVE READING

Karen felt like a very sensitive person, but very controlled. The kind of person who had all of the socks in her drawer in line and organized by length. I also saw that Karen had a hard time making mistakes. She seemed driven to perfection in every area of her life, whether it was work, home, cleanliness, and so on.

THE BODY

I looked at her head. Details, details, details! It seemed like details were very important to Karen. Her body seemed equally perfectionistic. Her muscles seemed tight and extremely well exercised. I saw a capacity to have problems with her thyroid hormone, particularly thyroid hormone T3. Her heart rate seemed slow. Her blood pressure seemed low. In her digestive tract, I saw red dots from her stomach to her esophagus, all the way to her mouth and gums. Her abdomen seemed bloated or distended, and I saw a problem with irregular bowel movements. Finally, I saw really low estrogen, low progesterone, and irregular menstrual cycles.

THE FACTS

Karen told me that her major problem was her digestion and constipation. She wasn't concerned about the fact that she didn't have periods. She was going to school to be a nutritional counselor. In fact, she was going to eventually ease her way out of a job as a CEO and become a nutritionist. Karen told me proudly, "I only get menstrual cycles if I weigh over a certain amount." Karen admitted that several people in her life were concerned about her weight and had labeled her anorexic and bulimic. Hearing this, I saw that the reading all made sense. The red-dotted pattern in her mouth, through her esophagus, all the way to her stomach was a form of inflammation. I asked Karen if she had induced vomiting in her life, and she admitted that from time to time, especially when she was stressed at work, she would feel calmer if she threw up. Karen admitted she had always been a perfectionist, dating back to when she was a ballet dancer as a teenager. She said proudly, "I'm used to being very detailed and regimented, and I don't really have much room for sloppiness." Karen just didn't understand how eating a raw diet or taking some nutritional supplements wouldn't fix her digestive problems.

THE BRAIN ADDICTED TO BEING THIN

We live in a culture where there is a lot of pressure to look good and perform perfectly. However, an addiction to being thin, eating disorders like anorexia and bulimia and the whole continuum between them, aren't just about people buckling under the social pressure to have the perfect body image. Yes, it's true that people look at magazines, movies, and other images to get a sense of, and then get confused about, what the ideal body type should be. Just as our body image can get distorted by past abuse, the visual circuits in our brain can get further manipulated and corrupted by magazines, social media, and TV.

Disrupted brain-body circuits for an addiction to being thin, however, aren't just environmental. There may be some genetic component or brain style to anorexia and bulimia, the most severe form of a brain disorder that's compelled to perpetual pursuit of being thin. If anorexia nervosa occurs earlier in your life, science tells us it's not necessarily precipitated by adverse events in your life. I don't know if all studies agree with that statement, but that's what most studies say. The later the onset of an eating disorder, the more likely it is associated with abuse, whether it's sexual abuse, physical abuse, or something else.

Overly restricting your food will ultimately have adverse consequences for your health. If you don't get enough food, it affects your energy needs and will affect your thyroid, heart, reproductive system, and bones, to list only a few organs, just as in the prior section we saw that eating too much food can lead to obesity, and inflammation in your body that increases your chance toward heart disease, stroke, diabetes, and so on. Bulimia, or the induction of vomiting, has its own set of complications, in that the acid from your stomach can burn the lining of the esophagus, your mouth, and your teeth, not to mention cause the loss of important electrolytes, potassium, and other chemicals that are important for a healthy heart rhythm. Many people with severe anorexia and bulimia, when their weight becomes dangerously low, end up having serious heart rhythm problems that are life-threatening.

Whether you are addicted to being thin or have the most severe form of food restriction—anorexia—or have bulimia or obesity, the entire spectrum of eating disorders has one thing in common: disordered eating. Disordered eating involves distorted self-image, self-esteem, and a need to medicate these feelings and thoughts with an eating addiction. Whether you're emaciated or obese, you try to compulsively control your self-love through thinness. Your brain is being hijacked by an addiction to food. How?

Consider the following. If in medical intuition we have seven emotional centers, each one being worth 14 percent of our daily life, food and eating, the third center, is supposed to involve only 14 percent of our attention. PERIOD. If during your day your thoughts and behavior involve looking for, planning, organizing, counting, measuring, weighing, and calculating nutrients, fat, protein, any and all components of what you put in your mouth as a food item, take note. This means that 86 percent of your life—that time that could be available for engaging with family, friends, work, hobbies, activism in your community, intellectual development, and spirituality—has been displaced by your singular obsession and compulsion. *That* is addiction. Now, you may argue, and it has been argued, that individuals with IBS, Crohn's, gluten enteropathy, and a variety of other digestive problems have to do just that: spend much of their day dealing with what they're going to eat, what they can tolerate, will this or that restaurant have food they can eat, and so on and so on. Though you might not want to call this addiction, you might certainly want to consider the fact that your health problem (believe me, I have something like this) has so taken over your life that it's displaced critical areas of function. If that's the case, like an addiction, your problem is not simply a digestive problem. Whether it's IBS, gluten enteropathy, or food allergies, if they have become so severe that they consume all your time, they have hijacked your life and, in medical intuition, become a seventh-center life-threatening issue. In essence, they begin to distort your brain, the areas for opiates, dopamine, reward, and relationship that will ironically starve you of life itself. And though you may get some relief from your cyclic changes in diet, whether it's gluten, dairy, or the systematic elimination of food intolerances, if increasing restrictions prevent you from "running with the herd," the people around you, and having a flexible life, relationships, and career, science suggests you're going to have more severe health problems than just digestion. Why? Because if your digestive tract problems lead you to solutions that involve not being able to eat around other people and adapt, then we know that at the very least, the lack of close friends and support in itself poses a similar risk to your health as if you smoked, drank, or were obese.[12]

THE SOLUTION

There are a variety of treatments for addiction to being thin or compulsive food restriction, depending on the severity of the behavior. Whether it's outpatient treatments with cognitive behavioral therapy, dialectical behavioral therapy, or inpatient treatment, all the treatments are similar: stabilize the weight, treat depression, anxiety, and past trauma, and identify the triggers that influence disrupted eating. In addition, we need to also identify health problems in the body. If a person has a compulsion to being thin or disordered eating, we need a thorough examination of the esophagus, stomach, teeth, gums, small and large intestines.

Does the person have reflux? Gastroparesis? Gluten allergies? Food intolerances? IBS, constipation, or other bowel problems? We need to check the bone density. If your body is very, very low in weight, you need to check levels of hormones, electrolytes, and potassium, as well as getting an EKG, a heart rhythm test, to make sure your heart has not been affected by weight loss.[11]

And if you have a compulsion to restrict food, whether anorexia or simply an obsession with being thin, consider if you are using food to treat mood and anxiety. If anxiety is your trigger for disordered eating, consider 5-HTP 100 milligrams three times a day, passion flower, or lemon balm. If you are trying to lower your weight to elevate your mood out of depression, you might want to consider SAMe or talk to a doctor about SSRIs. Some individuals who have bipolar disorder or other mood disorders may not do well on serotonin agents but may do better with mood stabilizers.

You can use yoga, aerobic exercise, and others as part of a balanced, total healing program. It's important to rehabilitate your self-image body, mind, and soul. However, especially if you have anorexia, consult with your counselor, coach, physician, or other practitioner on how often you should exercise. For some individuals, especially with a compulsion to be thin, or anorexia, overexercise is part of their extreme weight-reduction technique.

THE AFFIRMATIONS

Like all eating disorders in medical intuition, anorexia and bulimia have to do with self-esteem and responsibility. Self-esteem meaning deservability. So the first treatment Louise offers for these conditions is deservability treatment. Start by reading this affirmation paragraph in the mirror every day:

> I am deserving. I deserve all good. Not some, not a little, but all good. I now move past all negative, restricting thoughts. I release and let go of the limitations of my parents. I love my parents. I do not love their negative opinions or their limiting beliefs. I do not value any of their fears or prejudices. I no longer identify with limitations of any kind. In my life, I'm moving into a new space of consciousness where I am willing to see

myself differently. I am willing to create new thoughts about myself and about my life. I now prosper in a number of ways. The totality and possibility lies before me. I deserve a good life. I deserve an abundance of love. I deserve good health. I deserve to live comfortably and to prosper. I deserve joy. I deserve happiness. I deserve the freedom to be all that I can be. I deserve more than enough. I deserve all good. The universe is more than willing to manifest my new beliefs, and I accept this abundant life with joy and pleasure and gratitude, for I am deserving. I accept it. I know it to be true.

Deserving has nothing to do with having good. It has to do with our willingness to accept it. We need to allow ourselves to accept good whether we think we deserve it or not. So Louise also suggests this deservability exercise. Answer the following questions as best you can:

1. What do you want that you are not having? Be clear and specific about it.

2. What are the laws and rules in your home about deserving? What did they tell you—that you don't deserve, or you deserve a good smack? Did your parents feel deserving? Did you always have to earn in order to deserve? Did earning work for you? Were things taken away from you when you did something wrong?

3. Do you feel that you deserve? What is the image that comes up? Later when I earn it? I have to work first for it? Are you good enough? Will you ever be good enough?

4. Do you deserve to live? Why? Why not?

5. What do you have to live for? What is the purpose of your life? What meaning have you created?

6. What do you deserve? I deserve love and joy and all good, or do you feel deep down that you deserve nothing? Why? Where did the message come from?

Are you willing to let it go? What are you willing to put in its place?

Remember, these are thoughts, and thoughts can be changed. You can see that personal power is affected by the way we perceive our deservability. Try this treatment, but most simply, treatments are positive statements made in any given situation to establish new thought patterns and dissolve old ones.

Louise follows the exercise up with additional affirmations:

- Bulimia is about hopeless terror, a frantic stuffing and purging of self-hatred. The affirmation is "I am loved and nourished and supported by life itself. It is safe to be alive."

- Anxiety is about not trusting the flow and process of life. The affirmation is "I love and approve of myself. I trust the process of life. I am safe."

- Menstrual cycle problems that often occur with eating disorders have to do with anger at the self, hatred of the female body. The affirmation is "I love my body. I love what I see. I rejoice in my femaleness. I love being a woman."

III. ALCOHOL ADDICTION

Besides food and cigarettes, alcohol is one of the leading addictions. Almost everyone knows someone in their family who was called "the alcoholic," the one passed out at the wedding. In any major city, we see thousands of homeless people who are in various stages of the mental and physical aspects of alcoholism, and perhaps that more visible face of this addiction may make it hard for us to admit when we or a loved one have this illness. For decades, perhaps centuries, alcohol addiction had a stigma; we didn't talk about it until a marriage was falling apart, a family was torn apart, someone had gone financially bankrupt, lost their job, or had serious legal problems.

After alcohol has disintegrated the fabric of one's life, it tends to, organ by organ, deteriorate the body as well. Whether it's ulcers, cirrhosis of the liver, anemia and bleeding disorders, infections, bone fractures, seizures, pneumonia, nutritional deficiencies, violent behavior, suicide, or dementia, extreme use and abuse of alcohol has catastrophic effects on one's life and the lives of everyone around one. Drinking alcohol over a certain level increases your risk for a variety of cancers as well, including colon, breast, liver, esophageal, gastric, and others, not to mention your risk for heart disease and stroke. So, even if we don't have a problem with alcohol abuse or disordered use, we all need to be vigilant about alcohol's effects on our life and others'.

Do the following statements and symptoms apply to you?

MIND SYMPTOMS

- You tend to drink beer, wine, whisky, or hard liquor to calm your nerves or lift your spirit.

- You have daily emotional and physical cravings to drink.

BEHAVIOR SYMPTOMS

- You use alcohol to get to sleep at night.

- You find yourself drinking larger amounts than you intended, such as drinking more drinks than you planned or finishing the entire bottle.

- You can't take part in social activities unless you drink.

- A great deal of your time is spent obtaining, using, or recovering from alcohol.

- Every week, empty bottles add up and you try to discard them anonymously.

- You've failed at some responsibility at school, work, or home because of alcohol—or so someone has told you.

- You've had to drink more and more to get the desired effect or to feel intoxicated.

- When you stop drinking, you get jittery and you can't get to sleep.

- You've had the following problems: osteoporosis, libido problems, ulcers, gastritis, elevated liver enzymes, cirrhosis of the liver, fatty liver, weight gain, pancreatitis, aspiration pneumonia, blackouts, seizures, or memory problems related to alcohol use; a brain injury due to an accident associated with your alcohol use; or two or more arrests for operating a vehicle under the influence of alcohol.

- You've tried several times to Cut back on your alcohol use, but you always end up going back to your former pattern.

- When someone asks you to cut down on your alcohol use, you get Annoyed.

- You feel Guilty when you drink.

- When you get up in the morning, as soon as you open your Eyes, you drink just a little alcohol to start the day.

If alcohol is an issue in your life or a loved one's life, consider the following story.

LINDA: I DON'T HAVE A PROBLEM WITH ALCOHOL, REALLY

Linda, 54, called me because she was having concerns about her health.

THE INTUITIVE READING

When I first read Linda, her mind felt very anxious, like a gerbil frenetically moving around and around and around on one of those wheels. Whether it was irritable, restless, or panicky, her mind seemed to go in all directions at once. I could see Linda's primary problem was compulsion, doing the same thing over and over and not being able to stop. I could see her buying lots of useless items and not being able to stop, running up her credit cards. I could see her working herself into exhaustion. I could also see her compulsively rescuing people in her family.

THE BODY

Once again, I could see Linda having a hard time stopping the thoughts from going around and around in her mind. Did she have difficulty stabilizing her thyroid hormone levels because of an autoimmune problem? I wondered whether or not her doctors were concerned about cholesterol and triglycerides. Intuitively, I could see that a lot of Linda's problem centered on the middle of her body, though. There seemed to be inflammation where her esophagus and stomach came together. There seemed to be fat collections in her liver, and I could see that she had problems with blood sugar. I wondered whether or not addiction ran in her family, whether it was alcohol, prescription medicines, or gambling.

THE FACTS

Linda told me she had problems with depression. She had been treated for years with stimulants for ADHD, but now her doctors wondered if she had bipolar disorder, because she went on shopping sprees, compulsively spending. At times, Linda had used alcohol and oxycodone to settle her nerves, and numerous times she had quit. Since menopause, she'd started to drink a little wine at night to get to sleep. Lately the doctors were concerned because she had reflux and elevated liver enzymes, and they wanted her to quit drinking altogether. Linda told me that nobody had any addiction in her family, other than the fact that her father gambled and her mother had to work two jobs to pay off the debts.

THE SOLUTION

Even though alcohol has become entrenched in our culture, in that it can be part of every meal, ceremony, or even religious observance, if it starts to affect your physical, emotional, or financial health, then alcohol is a problem in your life. In a way, then, it really doesn't matter how much you use or how frequently you drink. If you have to continue to drink, if you are compelled to use alcohol despite adverse effects on your health, your relationships, and your job, it's an addiction.

According to the World Health Organization, alcohol is the fifth greatest contributor to the global burden of disease. Alcohol is the number one form of addiction, behind food and cigarettes. And it's expensive, in that excessive use of alcohol increases our chance toward heart disease, stroke, dementia, and cancers, especially cancers of the digestive tract and breast cancer. People who have depression or bipolar disorder are more likely to try to treat their own mood with alcohol, not to mention other substances. At first it will feel as if the alcohol is helping you get to sleep, or in fact calming your "nerves." However, over time, alcohol actually depresses your mood and disrupts your sleep cycles.[13] Often people switch from alcohol and go to another drug to "calm their nerves" or get to sleep, especially in menopause. At many Alcoholics Anonymous (AA) meetings you can find dozens of donuts in the back of the room or people smoking outside in a nicotine haze. And although people are stopping one addiction, alcohol, they're replacing it with another, nicotine or food. Six of one, half a dozen of the other. Apples or oranges. Whatever metaphor you want to use, you have to figure out how to regulate the emotion you're medicating with addiction or how to handle anxiety, depression, ADHD, or other brain disorders without using an addiction to medicate those problems. Otherwise, you'll find you have multiple problems with your mind and multiple addictions, with spiraling deleterious effects. Whether you drink too much, eat too much, smoke too much marijuana, spend too much, or work too much, in the end all these cumulative addictions will distort the way you relate to your family, mate, work, children, and society in general.

THE TREATMENTS

So what DO you do if you have anxiety and depression and alcohol seems to work? If you find yourself using alcohol or, as in the previous sections, food or other substances compulsively to medicate your mood, stop. You have choices. First, go to your nearest mental health center and find an addiction professional. They will help assess you for "dual diagnosis," and what problems you have with anxiety and depression, ADHD, and other problems along with a possible addiction. There are a variety of ways that practitioners evaluate for depression, anxiety, and ADHD that is compounded by alcohol or other addictions. First, the counselor uses an "inventory" of sorts (I'm not going to give you the name of the inventory, because they're always changing). These inventories help identify to what degree you have a problem with alcohol, but often they can be applied to marijuana, cigarettes, cocaine, gambling, shopping, collecting, fill in the blank. You name the addiction, you can apply this inventory to it. But for this section we're just going to form these questions about alcohol. Ask yourself the following:

1. Do you use alcohol in larger amounts or over a longer period of time than you intend?

2. Do you have a difficult time cutting back or controlling your use of alcohol?

3. Is much of your life spent in activities around using alcohol or recovering from its effects?

4. Do you have a craving or strong desire often to use alcohol?

5. Does drinking alcohol often cause you to fail at your major responsibilities, as in work, school, home, or relationships?

6. Does your alcohol use cause arguments or problems?

7. Have you avoided certain work or recreational activities because it would prevent you from using alcohol?

8. Have you used alcohol despite it being physically hazardous?

9. Have you continued to use alcohol despite it having adverse physical or psychological consequences, that is, do you have a physical diagnosis where the doctor tells you that continuing to drink might injure your health?

10. Have you had to drink more and more to get the same effect?

If you have answered yes to at least two of these, then it is a significant suggestion that you have a problem with alcohol (or whatever it is that you use compulsively). Your addiction treatment professional will help you go through that list, and perhaps it may be important for you to bring your significant other or another honest friend who is not an employee—a friend who is not afraid to be honest who really cares for you. If you find that you do have a problem, understand that sometimes, and I'm not trying to give you platitudes here, it's difficult to even come to grips with the fact that there is a problem, let alone identify the variety of solutions that will work and then actually engage effectively in the solutions.

ANSWERS FOR ADDICTION

There's a wide variety of 12-step programs that can help with a variety of addictions:

- Alcoholics Anonymous
- Narcotics Anonymous
- Gambler's Anonymous

- Sex Addicts Anonymous

- Codependents Anonymous

The list is endless.

Some people can be helped with a 12-step group alone, but if you have dual diagnosis, addiction with depression, ADHD, or anxiety, it's important that you simultaneously get treatment for your other disorder, whether it's medication, nutritional supplements, or cognitive behavioral therapy.[14] In the case of alcohol, your doctor will find out what nutritional deficiencies you may have. People with severe alcohol use may not get enough B12 and folate. They may in fact develop a thiamine deficiency and develop some problems in the memory centers of the brain. This is not necessarily a rare and obscure syndrome, because it occurs in 12.5 percent of all alcoholics.[15] There are a variety of other long-term changes that can occur in people with severe alcohol use. They can develop ulcers in their stomachs, reflux, gastritis, not to mention cirrhosis of the liver, as well as peripheral neuropathy, a disturbance of weakness and numbness, pain and tingling in their feet. Unfortunately, these symptoms can sometimes get worse even after the alcohol use stops. Alcohol use can cause other disorders over time, including muscle pain.

So it's important if you do have an addiction to also evaluate your nutrition. In the case of alcohol intake, this chemical causes a malabsorption of vitamin B1, thiamine, vitamins A, D, B6, E, and folate. So if you are actively in the throes of this addiction, it's important to take a multivitamin, even though, taking one, you might not be absorbing it, because of the alcohol you are also taking. Taking coenzyme Q10, 400 to 600 milligrams a day, might help protect your heart, not to mention your breasts. Alcohol is notorious for causing both cardiovascular problems and breast cancer.[16] There are medicines to help get over the addiction as well. There are a variety of medicines that people have used to help individuals maintain sobriety, including Zoloft, naltrexone, and by the time you're reading this book, probably others.[17] It's important not to be judgmental or critical about what your unique path is to becoming sober. What's important is that you actually do stay away from the substance you're addicted to and start to learn the emotion you cover up with that substance. That is, you achieve sobriety with support.[18]

THE AFFIRMATIONS

Often people who use alcohol have problems with PTSD, anxiety, insomnia, or guilt, not to mention the physical disorders that the alcohol may either medicate or cause. So, when doing affirmations, it's important to use not just affirmations for the addiction, but affirmations that apply to the symptoms you're having. In this case, the physical symptoms would be high cholesterol, cardiovascular disease, lower back pain, and carpal tunnel syndrome. (See Appendix B.)

Louise offers the following affirmations:

- For alcohol dependence, the thought is "What's the use?" There's a feeling of futility, guilt, inadequacy, self-rejection. The affirmation is "I live in the now. Each moment is new. I choose to see my self-worth. I love and approve of myself."

- For post-traumatic stress disorder and anxiety, there's a problem with trusting the flow and process of life. The affirmation is "I love and approve of myself. I trust the process of life; I am safe."

- For insomnia, fear, and guilt, the affirmation is "I lovingly release the day and I slip into peaceful sleep knowing tomorrow will take care of itself."

- High cholesterol reflects clogging the channels of joy, because we fear accepting joy. The affirmation is "I choose to love life. My channels of joy are wide open. It is safe to receive."

- For lower back pain, which relates to fear of money and lack of financial support, the affirmation is "I trust the process of life. All I need is always taken care of."

- For sciatica, which has to do with being hypercritical, fear of money and the future, the affirmation is "I move into my greatness and good. My good is everywhere. I am secure and safe."

- For carpal tunnel syndrome, the thought pattern is anger and frustration at life's seeming injustices. The affirmation is "I now choose to create a life that is joyous and abundant. I am at ease."

- And, finally, for pain in general, the feeling is aching, for love, longing to be held. The affirmation is "I love and approve of myself. I am loving and lovable."

IV. Multiple Addictions

If addiction is a process in which the networks in our brain for reward spiral out of control, many people in science and medicine have suggested that addiction is a disease. We have a network in our brain for reward and satisfaction. If you have a genetic susceptibility for that area to get hijacked by a substance like alcohol, science says that you have a susceptibility in your brain to be "addicted" to multiple substances as well.

In fertilization, we have an egg at the beginning of life, and sometimes the egg divides and you get twins or triplets—multiple births. But the original being was a single egg. Similarly, addiction is one problem, which, if left uncontrolled, can divide into twin addictions, or triplets, or quadruplets, or quintuplets. So first, as in the second case in this chapter, you may find yourself having a problem with overeating. That's the first addiction. And then in perimenopause, to get to sleep, if you're genetically susceptible, you may find yourself abusing alcohol. And when that starts to spiral out of control and a doctor suggests that you stop drinking because of digestive problems and a suspicious mammogram, you try to stop by going to AA. So now you have twin addictions: food and alcohol. You try to avoid the donuts in the back of the meeting room, because that's your other addiction, right? However, on your way out, you smell the cigarette smoke. Remembering your cigarette habit in high school, you find yourself calming your nerves with first one cigarette and then another. At first convincing yourself that you're only a casual smoker because you never buy a whole pack of cigarettes, you just borrow them, after you a while you realize that your "borrowing" has escalated to three packs a day. Now you have triplet addictions: eating, alcohol, and smoking. And though, allegedly, your eating and alcohol are in "remission," your smoking is not. Why? Because the nucleus accumbens and ventral tegmentum, the brain areas for reward and satisfaction, are still aberrantly out of control.

Finally, your doctor catches on, notes you have reflux, smells the cigarette smoke, and tells you to stop smoking. You do, and after a year of sobriety from "triple" addiction, you have to have surgery on your back for a prolapsed disc. Postoperatively, the doctor gives you a pain medicine, oxycodone. You find it's fabulous. Not only does it make your mood feel wonderful—better than it has in years—but you can get to sleep better than you have in what seems decades. When you return to your doctor to refill the prescription in the second or third month after surgery, you are stunned. Your doctor refuses to refill it because he says you have a history of addiction and you have to see an addiction specialist. You go back to the original addiction specialist you saw for alcohol, your first addiction, and that astute professional counts your multiple addictions that have now become not twins, not triplets, but quadruplets. You're addicted to food, alcohol, cigarettes, and now opiates. If you think this is rare, think again. Addiction is addiction.

In essence, there really is no such thing as multiple addictions. If you're addicted to one thing, one substance, your brain style gives you a capacity to be addicted to everything. If you're addicted to one thing, like alcohol or food, you have an addictive brain tendency. They used to call this the addictive personality. Of course, the personality is a byproduct of your brain.

Take the inventories in the previous sections and apply them to any substance you use in your life that has taken over your life like weeds in a garden. Apply the CAGE questions. Have you tried to Cut back on X? Do you get Annoyed when someone tells you that you're getting "out of control" with X? Do you feel Guilty when yet again you are compulsively engaging in X? And finally, the moment you wake up and open your Eyes, is X one of the first things you think about and do? Yes, like a cage, your substance or behavior, whether it's food, alcohol, smoking, gambling, spending, sex, collecting Beanie Babies, shopping on eBay, whatever—it has caged you in, hijacked the circuits in your brain, and taken over your life. Consider the following story.

MARK: A SHELL GAME OF ADDICTIONS

Mark, 41, called me for help because his health was a merry-go-round.

THE INTUITIVE READING

When I first did his reading, Mark felt like he fidgeted, fidgeted, fidgeted, fidgeted. *I* fidgeted when I was doing the reading. My mind went from one thing to another, so I realized that his mind couldn't stay on one train of thought. He felt charismatic, attractive, and charming, but didn't seem to stay in a relationship for very long. Although he seemed to have a good heart, I had a hard time seeing him being in a job for very long or being able to show up on time. Mark felt like one of those wheeler-dealer kinds of people who like to take risks. It felt like the latest huge risk had somehow failed and he'd lost a huge amount of money.

THE BODY

It felt like Mark had problems with focus and attention and was highly distractible. Did he crave stimulation? Chemical stimulants? Environmental stimulants? Whatever it was, he was "stimulus-bound." I saw dark clouds in his lungs. Did Mark smoke, or was he around somebody else who smoked? The blood vessels in his body felt stiff. I wondered over time whether he would have problems with blood pressure. I saw that red-dotted pattern in his esophagus and stomach area. I wondered whether or not he ran around with people who had addictions, whether it was alcohol or other chemicals. I saw changes in opiates in his body, and I saw changes in the motility of his bowel.

THE FACTS

Mark laughed when I told him he was distractible and craved stimulants. He told me he had a long history of attention deficit disorder and had used Ritalin for years as a child. He stopped taking the Ritalin and then started smoking at age 13. Despite the fact that he developed asthma, he still continued smoking cigarettes. After quitting high school and getting his GED, Mark moved to Vegas and found out he was better at gambling than working a nine-to-five job. He lost more than one marriage as a result of the ups and downs of his gambling debts. He said, "You have to stay ahead of the game. There's only some people who can make a living at gambling, and I'm one of them." Having played football in high school, he also did well in the Internet football pools and other forms of gambling. An old football injury in his knee followed by several knee surgeries got him hooked on pain meds— oxycodone and opiates.

THE SCIENCE OF MULTIPLE ADDICTION

Whether it's nicotine, oxycodone, or stimulants like cocaine, all addiction tends to affect the area in the brain for opiates, the area for reward, motivation, and drive.[19] Cigarettes are one of the most difficult addictions to successfully manage, although alcohol and eating are right up there. Why is it so hard to quit smoking? We have educational programs explaining the positive aspects of quitting. People know how to use patches or medicines to quit. So why is it so hard? Functional MRI studies show that nicotine alters responses in the brain to how we experience reward. Smokers' brains respond less to money, to non-drug sources of reward, but they respond more to nicotine. Somehow the brain reward areas for work, relationships, have been taken over, strongly hijacked by this drug. So it's really hard for educational programs alone to have much effect if your brain has been chemically enshackled by a substance like cigarettes or nicotine. Over time, one could say the same whether the drug of choice is alcohol, cocaine, gambling, or anything, really.

Why are some of us addicted and others not? There must be some genetic, biochemical, or temperamental difference in how people's brains process reward, whether it's from drugs, food, gambling, rescuing, money, relationships, what have you. People who are casual smokers show a greater reward in their brain for money and relationships than they do for cigarettes, but not people who are addicted to cigarettes. In Chapter 4, we're going to talk about learning styles and learning disabilities. What's important to understand is that all of us have a unique genius, some area in our brain that works incredibly efficiently. The downside is that each and every one of our brains has an area that doesn't work so efficiently. In Mark's case, his attention areas don't work as well and it may be that he's craving stimulus because, in a way, environmental stimulus, such as taking risks, drives the adrenal gland to produce epinephrine, like dosing himself with the Ritalin he used to use as a child. Your brain stem produces norepinephrine and stimulants, similar in a way to taking medicines like Ritalin, cocaine, and others. Whether it's drama, chaotic relationships, skydiving, high-risk investments, or any high-wire behaviors we may engage in, they may provide the neurotransmitters that help a person with ADHD pay attention and organize thoughts and life. Nicotine is a stimulant too. Many of my friends that are so ADHD they are off the charts, after they've quit smoking, they have nicotine gum all over their house!

You cannot ignore the brain you have. Otherwise, you will find out that your life has been shaped by the compensatory strategies of addiction. Initially, addiction might medicate your brain away from depression, anxiety, attention deficit, and so on, but over time, those brain pathways can't stay medicated on a specific dose that you use of your "addictive substance." You'll require more and more food, alcohol, cigarettes, gambling, rescuing, sex, chaos and drama, and so on, and over time your attempts to medicate your unique brain style to function will have health effects on you and everyone around you. In this book so far we've learned to identify our unique mood circuits, depression, irritability, anxiety, and now addiction. In the chapters ahead we'll talk about learning styles, learning disorders, spirituality, and intuitive ability. In all these areas there's a plus side to having that unique brain challenge, in that you get some savant or exaggerated "genius" gifts, if only you can learn to soothe, support, or "medicate" the downside.

So understand that your addiction is part and parcel of you trying to self-medicate that part of your brain that gives you a little bit of difficulty.[20]

Getting to Know Your Brain

One of the ways I get to know how a person's brain is organized is by asking them what substances they've used, been attracted to, or abused. I ask them what street drugs they've taken, enjoyed, or had bad reactions to. Many people are a little embarrassed when I ask them this question because they're getting ready to be pre-shamed. I'm not shaming them. I know that all of us use substances to medicate ourselves. Diet soda, fried dough, wine, cocaine, marijuana, LSD, and so on: our bodies and brains know what we need biochemically, at least in the moment.

If you crave, oh, I don't know, roller coasters, sugar, chocolate (that's me, of course), it tells me something about the dopamine and stimulus areas of your brain. That is, you need more stimulation, whether it's from the point of view of attention, mood, or otherwise. If, on the other hand, caffeine drives your nerves up a wall and instead you really like Xanax or alcohol, then that tells me that you have a GABA issue and you may have concerns about anxiety and insomnia.

With a lack of understanding of the long-term effects of medicating yourself with stimulants, drugs, gambling, and so on, you may seek these substances for momentary relief of brain symptoms.

And though you will numb depression and anxiety and escape the pain of ADHD or dyslexia or some problem with learning (we'll learn about that in Chapter 4), you're more likely to develop an addiction. And, by not understanding and learning how to better heal your mind with medicine, intuition, and affirmations, you will not be learning how to use your whole mind. What do I mean by *whole mind*? By numbing yourself away from your moods, irritability, and panic, and learning unbalanced ways of dealing with attention deficit disorder, dyslexia, and so on, you are less likely to learn to use both your intellect and your intuition, that is, your whole mind. Thus the title of this book: *Heal Your Mind: Your Prescription for Wholeness through Medicine, Affirmations, and Intuition*.

Look at each and every chapter of this book. Now, if you are using substances or behavior to "run away from" depression, anger, panic, you are in essence also blotting out or numbing your intuition. You will also, by using alcohol, cigarettes, food, and other behaviors, be numbing yourself to potential opportunities for love and joy, whether they're in family, intimate relationships, work, or connection to the divine. When it comes to the chapters ahead, if you have difficulties with paying attention, learning, memory, or finding peace spiritually, then clouding your brain and body with addictions like alcohol, food, smoking, gambling, and so on, equally prevents you from accessing all of your intelligence and intuition. In the remaining chapters of this book, we're going to help you learn how to use your unique brain for learning, paying attention, and memory, so you can access all of your intelligence—both your intellect and your intuition.

The Solution

There are a number of solutions that you can use for addiction. You may think that you have to have someone point out which of your substances or behaviors are addictions: rescuing, gambling, food, and so on. For smoking, there are a variety of nicotine lozenges, patches, Wellbutrin, the list is endless. Acupuncture helps us support our brain and our body to remove a substance from our life and eliminate cravings as well as withdrawal symptoms.[21]

In addition to twelve-step programs, cognitive behavioral therapy and motivational therapy can also have a dramatic effect on "poly-substance abuse," but especially opiate abuse, whether it's heroin, oxycodone, or any other opiate.[22] If you have physical pain that's complicating your opiate use, it's important to have a multidimensional treatment plan. Opiate dependency is very complicated. It requires a treatment team: a psychiatrist, pain management specialist, physical therapist, psychotherapist, acupuncturist, massage therapist, or neuromuscular therapist. Along with that, you might want to consider having a nutritionist, homeopathic doctor, osteopathic doctor, or naturopathic physician complete your team to achieve optimal balance between pain control and improved functioning.

Some people also consider using medicines to maintain sobriety. This area is very controversial. Physicians and laypeople often are critical of replacing one drug dependency with another. Specifically, when it comes to opiate abuse and addiction recovery, some medicines, which shall remain nameless, have been prescribed to prevent people from using heroin or oxycodone on the street. However, some of these "prescribed medicines" have themselves been sold on the street by a process called drug diversion. Individuals have learned to crush up the pills, shoot them, and get high, as if they were using heroin or oxycodone, thus circumventing the whole point of the medicine, which was to maintain some semblance of drug sobriety. Therefore, some individuals who want to deal with their opiate addiction choose not to use prescription medicines at all, to prevent reusing.[23]

THE AFFIRMATIONS

Louise tells smokers that quitting is their decision to make. There is no right or wrong involved. She tells them, "Smoking came into your life at the right time, and it will leave at the right time in a perfect way." And she offers specific affirmations for the thought patterns for all the health problems that are associated with any addiction, whether with lungs, bowels, or otherwise. So beyond the affirmations below, if you have physical problems associated with your addiction, go to the back of the book and look for those health problems in Appendix B. If you have depression, anger, or anxiety, which is why you're using the addictive substance in the first place, go to those parts of the book and follow the solutions there.

- For lung problems, COPD, or emphysema, the thought pattern is that you're not worthy of living. The affirmation is "It is my birthright to live fully and freely. I love life. I love me."

- For respiratory problems, fear of taking in life fully, the affirmation is "I am safe. I love my life."

- For problems with pain meds or pain in general, the problem is guilt. Guilt always seeks punishment. The affirmation is "I lovingly release the past. They are free and I am free. All is well in my heart now."

- For constipation, the side effect that you experience from pain meds, the thought pattern is refusing to release old ideas, being stuck in the past. The affirmation is "As I release the past, the new, fresh, and vital enter. I allow life to flow through me. And all is well."

ALL ROADS LEAD TO ADDICTION

I have been a physician and a medical intuitive for over 30 years. I have heard and seen the most amazing cases: individuals whose bodies and lives are wondrous, filled with miracles, but also have a common thread, and that is that we're all just trying to do the best we can. The scientist in me often remembers the most unique and profound stories. In medicine we call those not the "horses" but the "zebras." So since my area has always been the brain, I've always been fascinated by the unique spiritual encounters people have had through brain disorders. I've often been enthralled by the remarkable symptom constellations that people have had, unique syndromes as in Oliver Sacks's book *The Man Who Mistook His Wife for a Hat*. Consider the following example, in which the details have been changed so it's not one individual. If you think you recognize yourself in this story, think again. It's an *example*.

When I was a resident, all the other physicians in the hospital would send me a patient if he or she had a unique, odd combination of brain disorders. The more peculiar, the more likely to become a "Mona Lisa patient." One day a patient came into my office and said, "The angels. Make them stop it!" Then in exquisite detail she proceeded to describe how every evening at the same time, a group of angels would come in through her kitchen door, banging their wings against the kitchen cabinets, and rifle through all her mail piled up on the kitchen table. The patient looked up at me with complete seriousness. "It's a federal offense to go through someone's mail. Make them stop."

Thinking about how people in the New Age movement spend millions of dollars a year to see angels, talk to angels, do everything "angel," I found it interesting that angels to this woman were an aversive phenomenon. So I asked her, "Have you ever tried to talk to them? Most people would love to have an angel or two visit them. Right?"

She looked up at me quizzically. "Not if they're going through your mail."

I asked the woman how long this had been going on. Was it her whole life? She said no, it was only in the last six months. In neuropsychiatry, you have to look "under the hood"—you have to look in the brain for a disorder. I decided to look at a specific area of the brain, the temporal lobe. Its normal function is for spirituality, but sometimes when a person has an illness there, exaggerated perception and reception for spirituality result. So we did an MRI and found that in fact the woman had a temporal lobe glioma in her right brain. (You will learn in Chapter 6 that the right brain is the chief area for spirituality and emotion and the temporal lobe specifically is the area with which one perceives the divine.) The patient agreed to the surgeon's suggestion to take the tumor out, because if that's what it would take for the angels to stop going through her mail, she was all for it.

Two months later, the patient returned to my office all healed. Fabulous! She was thrilled, because nobody had come in her kitchen door lately except her friends, and none of them had wings. Her mail was safe from intrusions. All was right in the patient's world.

But two months after *that,* the patient came back and she was mad as hell. She said, "The angels are back, and I called the police and they're not taking me seriously."

I was stunned, because they'd taken out the tumor, the "offending agent" in her brain that was eliciting this disturbing phenomenon for her. She was also on an anticonvulsant, a medicine that would stabilize any electrical charges that might result from the surgery. There was really no medical reason why she should be having "angel visitors."

I asked her for a list of medicines she was taking, everything she was putting in her mouth, because I was thinking perhaps she might be having a kind of altered state of consciousness, brain fog, delirium. She happily gave me a list of her medicines, which included a large dose of marijuana. Marijuana smoked six to eight times a day. She had taken it in high school, and had recently resumed using it because it helped her relax. And it just so happened that the escalation of her marijuana use and abuse coincided with the frequency of the angels' visits. When I suggested to her that she might consider stopping marijuana, that it might be creating brain fog and delirium, she got mad, saying, "People are always trying get me to cut back on my marijuana use. Why should I listen to you? I don't listen to anybody else." And she walked out in a huff. Suffice it to say, she continued to use marijuana (and, I might add, other illicit drugs) despite adverse medical consequences.

The phrase I'd like to leave you with is "All roads lead to addiction." In the most elegant cases, in the most common cases and the most unusual ones, in almost every situation, one can find addiction. Addiction is not unique. If you think it doesn't affect your family, think again. If you think you're in a special situation in which it doesn't touch your life—if you think you're unique— well, you know what AA says: they call it the disease of terminal uniqueness.

Chapter 4

BRAIN AND LEARNING STYLES

Do you have trouble paying attention to details? Do you have difficulty following someone who's telling you a story, or giving you a set of directions, or having a lengthy conversation? Does your mind trail off when someone is speaking to you or when you're watching a movie or a TV program? Do you have trouble finishing work, whether at school or in your workplace? Do you easily get sidetracked by what's going on around you? Do you lose things you need for an activity, whether it's your purse, wallet, keys, eyeglasses, paperwork, and so on? Do you have difficulty reading books or even paragraphs in magazines and newspapers because it requires so much effort? When you were in school, did you try to avoid classes that involved writing papers because you tended to have problems with grammar, syntax, and paragraph organization? Are you socially nervous or anxious? Do you tend to enjoy nature, machines, or technology more than people? Has it always been difficult for you to comprehend people's unspoken emotion, their facial expressions, emotional nuance and subtlety?

If you have had a lifelong struggle with any of these symptoms, your brain may be structured differently from most. The way you reason, problem-solve, experience, perceive, learn, and remember the world, not to mention communicate with and relate to others, may be different. However, the way your brain is uniquely constructed may have, in the past and in the present, made it difficult for you to function in your family, school, and work and handle finances and relationships.

Everybody to some degree has one or two unique subtleties that make their brains different. Since my Ph.D. program in behavioral neuroscience and neuroanatomy, many of my friends are neuropsychologists—those individuals who in fact evaluate brain styles and learning disorders. One neuropsychologist told me recently that Americans specifically have a difficulty with having a weakness in any cognitive area. She said they want to have superior scores on their IQ tests across the board, and if they have one or two dips in one score or another, they are crestfallen and think they have a disability. I looked at her, because I was crestfallen at some of my own scores. She said to me, in a practical tone, "You can't be good at everything. If you're human, you're just going to be better in some areas in your brain than others. It's not necessarily a disability. It's normal." So, if you have one or two of these symptoms, it's normal. So, maybe your mind trails off a bit when someone is giving a long-winded talk. Okay. Or maybe you're one of those people who loses their keys a lot. It doesn't necessarily mean you have ADHD or some other learning disability. It's only a problematic brain style if it makes it hard for you to function in your life, be it in work, school, relationships, or otherwise.

Somewhere between 3 percent and 20 percent of all people in our culture get labeled with a so-called learning disability. After all, we're one of those cultures that likes to put labels on people. Think about it. If 20 percent of all people have a disability, is it really a disability? Or is it just a different way of being normal, like, say, left-handedness? I prefer to think of "learning disabilities" as just a different way of being—a different style of brain.[1]

When I talk about learning, I'm not just talking about learning in school. Learning disabilities, in the sense that term has often been used, are not just about going to the resource room at school or getting extra tutoring. Learning difficulties don't go away when children become adults. Problems with acquiring new information—that is, learning—persist, because they involve having an unusual type of brain development. This doesn't just involve learning to read and write; it may involve acquiring the ability to socialize with other people. It's not about IQ level, either; an inability to learn may have nothing to do with your general level of intelligence. Someone can be very, very bright, but may not be able to demonstrate his or her intelligence in how he or she reads or writes. Unfortunately, for those individuals, their progress in high school and college may be hampered, not to mention in their careers, because most of the way we communicate with each other is through literacy.[2]

Many people who have been labeled as having "learning disabilities" actually aren't disabled at all. They end up having extremely successful lives. But if I slip and say "learning disability" or "learning disorder" in this chapter, understand that's just because everybody else does. If you've been diagnosed with ADHD, attention deficit disorder, the reading disorder dyslexia, and so on, you may not recognize how to handle your problem if I call it a "learning style difference," so bear with me.[3]

WAYS OF LOOKING AT BRAIN STYLES

Learning is a key part of our intuition. It's a specific part of our brain style. Everyone has intuition in one form or another, and it's born out of your unique brain style, whether it's attention or attention deficit disorder, being incredibly literary, having dyslexia, or a variety of other brain organizations. And though this chapter is about learning styles and their disorders, know that everyone has an area of genius and everyone has an area as a result that's not so well defined, that allows them to develop intuition. (More on this in Chapter 6.) Those areas that are not so refined may eventually be labeled as a learning disorder or some other problem.

How does one get a "learning disorder," or a different brain style, anyway? In people with dyslexia or attention deficit disorder, or any of the different learning disability diagnoses that are given out, what causes these disorders?

Sometimes, you can actually see structural differences in the brain. In other people, the ability to speak, read, write, or socialize just lags behind as their brains mature more slowly than others'. Some individuals have a different way in which their right and left brain connect. And if we grow up in an environmental situation where we're deprived, or there's chaos or drama, our brains may not learn as easily or effectively.[4]

No one knows why certain disorders are diagnosed more in women than in men, in girls more than in boys. For example, ADHD, attention deficit hyperactivity disorder, is more "common" in boys than in girls. Why is that? Is it because testosterone may influence brain development? Is it because our society is better at detecting attention problems in boys than in girls? Maybe. We do know that hormones have an impact on brain development. Elevated levels of androgens, that is, testosterone, influence left brain development for language. It has been found that elevated testosterone levels in critical periods of brain development may cause learning disorders in men.[5]

However, even though boys may be diagnosed with ADHD and dyslexia more often than girls, more recent studies show that girls may have different forms of dyslexia, and they also may be more able to compensate for or cover up their disorder thanks to how their brains are wired. So, you see, there are so many reasons why a person can develop a disorder that we cannot really say that any one factor causes it.

LEARNING STYLES AND MEDICAL INTUITION

What is the connection between your unique learning style, maybe even learning disability, and medical intuition? Simple. Intuition, at least by my definition, is the capacity to make a correct decision with insufficient information.[6] (This statement doesn't just come from me; it's based on some landmark studies by Antonio Damasio on the anatomy of intuition and decision making.) So when it comes to your brain and body style, in the areas where you have had problems—say, problems acquiring information (learning)—at times you have to fill in the gaps with intuition to function.

Say you have dyslexia, a left brain learning disability. When you've tried to read over the years, you may have adapted by learning a variety of methods for enhanced comprehension, but over time you realize your writing and reading are never going to be like everyone else's. Your brain is simply different. And whether you realize it or not, you use that other sense, intuition, to fill in the gaps when you read, to grasp what's written even though your unusual left brain is not picking it up. Similarly, people with ADHD have brains that are unique in how they perceive and take in the world. Whether they have difficulty with organization, planning, or distractibility, these individuals at times may make a lot of mistakes and actually get into trouble at work, in school, or in relationships. However, when it's absolutely critical, their intuition may swoop in to give them the pinpoint awareness and urgent focus required by the suffering of a loved one or an impending crisis.

Whether we have a learning disorder or not, we may develop a variety of health problems in our life. Even as we try to access the medical-intuitive meaning, the message that the pain behind these symptoms is giving us about our life or the life of a loved one, we also may feel that the health problem has disordered our life and hampered us in some ways. It's not so. Just like learning disorders, many health problems give us savant abilities, unusual intuitive capacities. How? That area where you have a health problem becomes part of your unique medical-intuitive network, a part that will for the rest of your life act up at times, signaling you that you need to "pay attention" and "read" a situation more clearly. That joint injury that turned to arthritis (first emotional center) will intuitively speak to you throughout your life whenever you don't feel safe and secure in a family. And that bout of diverticulitis or ulcerative colitis (third center)? For the rest of your life—even if you've been able to heal your digestion with nutritional supplements, herbs, medicines, and a variety of other remedies—when your work is making you feel awful, you will get that very familiar intuitive pang in your stomach. Medical intuition is a unique source of how we learn, remember, and make decisions in our lives.

THE ATYPICAL BRAIN

In Louise's first book, *Heal Your Body*, among the conditions and health problems listed, there's no listing for learning disability. There's no dyslexia, there's no ADHD in her book. Louise says that people with these labels are normal. Their brains have just developed differently.

There's a lot of support in the literature for this way of looking at learning disabilities. Some research scientists believe that instead of using multiple diagnoses for a laundry list of learning disabilities a person may have, we should just diagnose a person with "atypical brain disorder." Rather than writing up a laundry list, these scientists suggest we just look at each individual's learning style and describe exactly how they pay attention, read, write, and function socially. How do we do this? The best way is to give a person a full-scale neuropsychological assessment. We look at the whole person, the learning abilities and the disabilities. I might add that if a person has a rather dramatic learning disability, such as ADHD or dyslexia, the cognitive problems may distort testing to such a degree that standard IQ tests cannot effectively come up with an accurate IQ. A general, single IQ number does not apply to these people, because there's such discrepancy between the individual scores, and the score based on their weak area pulls all the other intelligence scales down. Hurrah! IQ simply doesn't apply to them. Lovely. That's why it's important not to put a number on a person, especially if they have a learning disability. What is more important to understand is how people process information, how they look at a problem and move to its solution.

A pioneer in this area is a neuropsychologist named Edith Kaplan, a mentor of mine in my M.D./Ph.D. program at Boston University School of Medicine. Edith developed something called the process approach to neuropsychology.[7] Edith couldn't stand batteries of tests to give a person an IQ number or find out what was wrong with his or her brain. She would say, "Batteries are for cars." Instead, Edith would take the same tests and, rather than just plunking the patient in front of the test and mechanically checking off what he or she got wrong or right, she would watch how the person approached the problem. By evaluating someone in this way, she didn't look at an attention *deficit*; she looked at how the person's attention *did* work. If she saw a person with dyslexia, she would see how the person approached the written word, and then she would be able to structure a program to help the person read better. She wasn't just interested in what was wrong with people's brains; she helped them find out how they could get to the right solution. So, today, when a person has a neuropsychological evaluation, we get an opportunity to look into how his or her brain functions, and then we can come up with a solution to help it function better.

Edith is essentially the mother of modern neuropsychology. She contributed much to what we know about developmental learning in the brain as well as, ultimately, how people can use creative alternative routes to process information. In my Thursday afternoon class with Edith, I remember in each session she would describe an early study by the *father* of neuropsychology, Norman Geschwind, whose work I cite in this book. It wasn't an ordinary class, because Edith wasn't an ordinary person. She obviously had a different way of processing information too. She was a creative, mercurial genius in her own right. Most of the classes in our Ph.D. program had a structure; they began at a certain time and ended at a certain time. But not Edith's. Edith's class would go on until Edith got winded. The class began at 4 P.M., and it would go on for hours. It could end at 9, it could end at 10, maybe 11. If any of us would doze off, Edith was famous for reaching into her purse, taking out a coffee candy, and flinging it at the student to keep them awake.

Did Edith have ADHD? Was she exhibiting some form of frontal executive function (you'll learn about that later)? *Yes!* But no one cared, because she was a genius. She was a productive, creative genius, and she was a revolutionary in her field, because that's what creative geniuses do. They learn to fit into a structure, and they transform it. And we felt lucky to be among the generations who were blessed to learn from her.

LEARNING DISORDERS AND AFFIRMATIONS

When it comes to the brain, Louise sometimes uses the metaphor of a switchboard or a computer. If you're concerned about having learning disabilities, whatever they may be, the affirmation is "I am a loving operator of my mind. I love myself just the way I am."

Many people look at learning disabilities as childhood diseases, but now we realize that's not true. We see learning disabilities in the same way modern neuropsychology does. We see that there is a place for everyone with every type of learning style. That each and every one of us can be given the tools to go beyond what some believe is a limitation. Although a term like *dyslexia* or *attention deficit disorder* or *Asperger's* or *autism* may lead people to think success is out of reach, this thought is neither accurate nor helpful. With modern approaches to neuropsychological assessment and neuropsychological remediation, all of us can learn to use our unique genius. However, Louise says that many of these false beliefs can diminish our capacity to appreciate the brain we were born with. If this situation is affecting you or someone you love, the affirmation is "A child is divinely protected and surrounded by love. We claim mental immunity."

When you're diagnosed with a learning disability, it may seem as if society is saying, "You're damaged. You can't reach all of your potential." Louise's affirmation for this is "I succeed in little things. I believe in my own power to change. Self-approval and self-acceptance are now the keys to my ability for positive change."

Many of us who have been labeled with learning disabilities begin to suffer from low self-esteem because we believe what people tell us, that we can't succeed. And we look around and we feel different and we feel that we can't deserve the success in life that the other people have, because they're not like us. So if you are that person with that diagnosis of ADHD, dyslexia, Asperger's, or autism, it's important to practice self-acceptance and also release yourself from other people's opinions. Louise has a treatment for this too. Her wonderful deservability treatment, which you read about in Chapter 3, begins with these affirmations: "I am deserving. I deserve all good. Not some, not a little, but all good. I now move past all negative, restricting thoughts. I no longer identify with limitations of any kind."

THE ALL IS WELL CLINIC

So maybe you've sailed through school, sailed through work, and you don't have any learning disorders. Maybe you have children and they're all Rhodes Scholars. They don't have learning disorders either. How could this chapter possibly help you? Because this chapter is about how to operate your brain for paying attention, using your right brain emotional relationship areas, not to mention learning how to skillfully manage life situations using your frontal lobe executive areas to be better organized, plan efficiently, and adapt to any circumstance. So, in essence, all of us can fine-tune every area of our brain to learn even more efficiently than it already does. By reading the following sections on each of the four brain disorders we are going to discuss (and there are others we aren't), even if you don't have that disorder, you can very much use the solutions to fine-tune your own brain for excellence.

On the other hand, if you've had struggles in school in the past, not to mention one job after another, walk right into the clinic and take a seat. Why? Maybe your boredom in school, inability to see the relevance of the assignments, or incapacity to feel comfortable in the social setting of school is the particular unique brain style you have that hinders your capacity to use all of your intellectual ability. If that's the case, then when you enter the workforce you may have trouble developing a career. It may be hard for you to make sense of written directions, not to mention oral assignments that are given to you in the office. You might have problems maintaining stable emotional footing in the midst of delicate politics in an organization. And finally, after a while, you may dispense with working in a job completely and find yourself year after year looking for that career that feeds your creative ability yet pays you well. You too may be having difficulty operating your unique intellectual style to function in the world of work and relationships.

I. ATTENTION DEFICIT HYPERACTIVITY DISORDER

Attention deficit hyperactivity disorder (ADHD) is a neurodevelopmental brain style that has been thought to occur at a higher rate in boys than in girls. Most people get this diagnosis when they're children. What you need to know is that this isn't necessarily a disease of children. It's a way in which you perceive the world.[8]

Our society is more attuned to picking up ADHD in boys than in girls. Wait a decade. You may find out that the incidence of these disorders is more equal between the genders than we've suspected.

So what is attention anyway? Paying attention involves multiple areas of the brain. Just as an orchestra requires multiple instruments to play, paying attention requires multiple channels in your brain to function. Whether it's the right brain, the parietal lobe, for divided attention, or the frontal lobe, the dorsolateral prefrontal cortex, for freedom from distraction, these two areas work together to help you focus on a task. The limbic system, the temporal lobe, helps you pay attention to things that are emotionally important to you; if you're depressed or anxious, your capacity to pay attention is far less. Last but not least, your brain stem produces neurotransmitters, serotonin, epinephrine, and dopamine, so if this area isn't working optimally, a neurotransmitter imbalance may make it hard for you to stay clear of brain fog and pay attention.

Since there are so many channels for attention, it makes sense that there are many types of medicines to help with disordered attention. I laugh when someone says to me that they think they have ADHD, so maybe they should go on Adderall. Really? Because they read a book that told them they were distracted, so they should be on something like Ritalin? Now that you know there are multiple areas in the brain that are involved with attention, you know the treatment for ADHD is not one size fits all.

So, if as you're reading this your attention is already trailing off, we need to find the unique strategy to help you fine-tune your brain's attentional circuitry. You can heal the attention in your mind with medicine, nutritional supplements, herbs, or therapy. Read on for the variety of solutions in the following story.

NANCY: DRIVING UNDER THE INFLUENCE OF DISTRACTION

Nancy called me for a reading because she was having trouble focusing and paying attention.

THE INTUITIVE READING

When I saw Nancy, it felt like her brain was different. She always had a hard time focusing and paying attention, but then when hormones started to hit her brain, it got even worse. I wondered whether or not she used carbohydrates to "help" her mind focus. I wondered whether addiction ran in her family. I had a hard time seeing stable work. In fact, I wondered whether Nancy had a long history of being undereducated and underemployed.

THE BODY

When I looked at Nancy's head, I myself had a hard time focusing and paying attention, as if my mind drifted away. The rest of her health didn't seem to be the issue, except her hormone cycle seemed to make her focus and attention worse. I wondered whether people in her family had thyroid problems. Were there problems with her neck? I wondered whether she'd had a series of accidents, because it seemed the muscles in her back were tight and could give her pain. I saw dark clouds in her lungs, which is usually the sign that someone around a person smokes. Were there red dotted patterns in her esophagus and stomach near her liver? I wondered whether addiction ran in her family to food, carbohydrates, alcohol, or stimulants.

THE FACTS

Nancy told me she had been diagnosed with ADHD. Instead of taking Ritalin when she was younger, she'd used stimulants—smoking, Diet Coke, Red Bull—to compensate. Other than a brief fling with cocaine in high school, Nancy felt that stimulants just weren't her bag. She said, "Oh, I also have diabetes, but the doctors said if I lose weight, I won't have to take insulin." Nancy told me that she could have gotten really good grades in high school and even gone to college, but she was "always bored."

On the other hand, she was not bored by relationships. She told me she had one chaotic and traumatic relationship after another. I asked her if that serial drama acted like a stimulant. Without that soap-opera, daytime-drama love life, would her mind and emotions feel dull? Nancy said, "Oh, my God, I never thought about that! I have relationship ADHD." She did, however, tell me she wanted to settle down and eventually have kids.

Nancy also admitted that she had always worked at low-wage jobs, but she wanted to get more training and become a paralegal. However, she wondered if her legal history, her problems with the law, would make that hard. She had had a series of alcohol-related car accidents and arrests. One accident was serious, and she'd suffered whiplash, which was the cause of that neck pain. Nancy wanted to know how she could go to school and improve her career if she couldn't pay attention and was always bored.

THE SOLUTION

Do you have trouble paying attention like Nancy? Do you often get bored? Do you use carbohydrates, Diet Coke, or relationship drama as a way of feeling more focused and alive? And, as in the last chapter on addiction, have you used stimulants or other substances addictively to sharpen your brain and focus, whether it's Red Bull, cigarettes, carbohydrates, and so on, ultimately with bad health effects? (See Chapter 3.) If so, there's a way to utilize your unique brain style for attention but not fry your brain and body with the stress that comes along with chaos and drama, not to mention the bad diet and addiction.

There is a unique wiring for a person who has ADHD. Whether it's a different right brain for divided attention or frontal executive function for freedom from distractibility, you have to figure out how to utilize all your circuits for attention to function in your family and your relationships, handle money, and pursue a vocation that utilizes your gifts and talents.

In addition, you have to figure out a way to use those right brain circuits for divided attention to balance what's going on in your emotional world with the feelings of those around you, as well as with information from intuition and the divine.

SLEEP

Regular sleep is critical for effective attention and memory. If you don't sleep, you can't pay attention. And get enough sleep in a bedroom that has no TV, I might add. If there are electronics in your bedroom, the constant beeping and signaling can interrupt your thoughts, not to mention your sleep. Sustained sleep at night is important for your hippocampus, the brain's memory areas, to create acetylcholine, a key neurotransmitter for attention and memory. If you are addicted to having technology in your bedroom, hire a friend to pry anything with a battery or a Bluetooth out of your sleeping chamber with the Jaws of Life. Even a wristwatch. Make sure you go to bed at the same time and get up at the same time every day, including weekends. Taking a multivitamin with B12 and folate can help your brain make serotonin, which is a key neurotransmitter for attention.

NUTRITION

There's a variety of other supplements that may be very effective for attention as well. They include but are not limited to:

- Ginkgo biloba 120 milligrams a day
- Omega-3 fatty acid (DHA) 1,000 milligrams three times a day
- Grapeseed extract 360 milligrams a day
- A multivitamin with B6 200 milligrams a day
- Folic acid 400 micrograms a day
- Vitamin B12 100 micrograms a day
- Amino acids: glutamine 500 milligrams a day and tyrosine 250 milligrams a day

These trace minerals, amino acids, and vitamins help your brain make neurotransmitters that stimulate your attention network. Also consider the following:

- SAMe, S-adenosylmethionine, helps your brain make dopamine and serotonin, key neurotransmitters for attention; take 400 milligrams two to three times a day on an empty stomach.

- Panax ginseng, 625 milligrams a day, doesn't just help with focus and attention; it is also an antidepressant.

- Gotu kola, also known as centella asiatica, is good for people who have anxiety and depression as well as attention problems. Typical dose is 600 milligrams three times a day.

- Small amounts of caffeine have a similar affect as Ritalin, so coffee and tea can be used in moderation. However, if you can sit still enough to meditate, for some it can be a better attention booster. (This isn't something I can do, so I'm not going to be a hypocrite.)

THE MEDICINES

By this writing, there will probably be many, many, many more medicines for ADHD because pharmaceutical companies are always coming out with more. You may or may not choose to use medicines. The gold standard for many years was Ritalin. However, using it is difficult if you have ADHD with anxiety. There are other similar substances, like Metadate, Concerta, Adderall, and others, that all essentially work on dopamine to help with focus and attention. Other medicines may help that are not nearly as addictive as Ritalin-like substances. These include Strattera as well as clonidine.

OTHER STRATEGIES

I would also suggest you consider getting a nonelectronic planner, one that uses pen and paper, to help you organize and plan your day. There's something about seeing something laid out in front of you that helps you organize your thoughts. Remember now, the frontal lobe area, site of organization, is an area that's often impacted with ADHD. This kind of planner helps substitute for your "working memory" or frontal executive function, which may not work so well if you have ADHD. Whether it's a Day-Timer, or a blackboard, or a peg board, you may need something external to you to get the organization, planning, and prioritization that is necessary when you're disorganized.

Someone who does cognitive behavioral therapy can also help you regulate your emotions and impulse control that can get you into trouble at work, with your family, and especially with finances.

THE AFFIRMATIONS

Yes, you may be using sweets, carbohydrates, caffeine, nicotine, alcohol, drama, chaos, environmental noise and busyness, to medicate your inattentive brain. However, a byproduct of excessive use of any of these substances or behaviors is also to numb your emotions, further distract you beyond what you realize, not to mention wreck your health and happiness. Louise has affirmations for many different addictions, depending on the substance you're addicted to. For example, the affirmation for sugar addiction would be "I now discover how wonderful I am. I choose to love and enjoy myself."

If you have ADD or ADHD and have the physical health fallout from your own attempts to compensate by using sugar, caffeine, nicotine, alcohol, drama, excessive exercise, and other things, look to the back of the book for health problems that may be byproducts of what you're using. Like every medicine has an effect and a side effect, how you're medicating your ADD may initially help but over time has a side effect. Consider the following ways you've treated yourself and illnesses that may have occurred. If you have the illness, go to the back of the book and do the affirmation associated with it.

- Sweets, carbohydrates—weight gain leading
  to diabetes

- Caffeine—heart palpitations, perhaps accelerating to
  heart problems

- Smoking of any substance, including nicotine—lung
  disease, asthma, and heart disease

- Excessive alcohol use—alcoholism

- Unstable relationships, chaos, unrelenting drama—uncontrollable up-and-down mood swings, PTSD

- Excessive exercise—lower back, knee, and other athletic injuries

- Excessive risk-taking—accidents, traumatic brain injury

II. DYSLEXIA

The next most common form of learning disability that people talk about is dyslexia. What is dyslexia? People with dyslexia simply have brains that are wired differently for language. Whether it's reading, speaking, writing, listening, or learning a language, your native language or someone else's, people with dyslexia find the process slow and inefficient, not to mention no fun.[9] People with dyslexia, especially if they're bright, may do fine in lower grades, but when they get to the higher grades and higher education, they may have trouble keeping up with the reading or the writing of papers. If you're particularly bright, you may compensate by spending more and more hours than other people on your assignments. Where one person may take a weekend to read a book, it may take you three weeks. After a while, you either avoid classes that involve reading books and writing papers or, worse yet, you simply don't finish your degree program.

So, if you find yourself having difficulty on multiple-choice tests, difficulty writing papers, difficulty remembering what you've read, you need to find out if you have a language-based learning disorder, that is, dyslexia. For people with this learning style, a problem with reading and writing is the stumbling block that prevents them from using all of their intellectual capacity to get ahead in life, in their vocation or their career.[10]

And if you have a brain that's pseudo-dyslexic, can you really "normalize" your brain? Probably not. When people with dyslexia get training to help them learn more efficiently, scientific studies do show that there is some normalizing of the brain areas for language. However, you really need to know that if you have dyslexia, you were simply born different. When you get tired or stressed, you will "decompensate," and it will be more difficult for you to read and write. If there is noise or distraction, it's going to be nearly impossible for you to read or write. So brace yourself, take a breath, and be patient with yourself. The important thing, as Louise says, is to love yourself just the way you are, but understand that you want to be the best you can be, especially, in this situation, with language. In fact, studies show that people with dyslexia have unique brains, with "warts" of sorts (brain cortical scars, especially in the left language areas). If you have dyslexia, you have to learn to love yourself "warts and all."[11]

Is this you? What do you do if you've gotten all the way through grade school, high school, college, and even an advanced degree program and you find out now you really do have a problem with dyslexia? During certain stages in your life, you may lose your usual tendency to compensate for your language disorder. Menopausal changes in estrogen may make it particularly hard for you to focus and ultimately tolerate the strenuous task that reading and writing is for you. There are numerous reasons why people may simply begin to realize that it's just too difficult to read the way they do.[12]

But the important thing to know is that it's never too late for help. If you find yourself in your 50s, with hormonal changes in your brain, feeling like you have a brain fog and those strategies you used to use to compensate for problems with reading and writing don't work anymore, now's the time to address your unique brain style for language, as in the following case.

OLIVIA: BEHIND THE EIGHT BALL AT WORK

Olivia, 49, called us for a reading because she was having trouble at work and making mistakes.

THE INTUITIVE READING

When I first looked at Olivia, I saw that she had always had a hard time feeling safe and secure in groups of people, whether it was in her family of origin, with her peers at school, or in her work environment. I saw that Olivia was very porous and sensitive. In fact, Olivia seemed to have a keen right brain intuitive sense, but somehow she wasn't using it, and her body and brain were letting her know this. She was very sensitive to the emotional pain and suffering of people around her, and I felt that it was affecting her emotional and physical health.

THE BODY

When I looked at Olivia's head, I saw problems with focus, attention, and distractibility. I could see that Olivia would try to focus on details, but after a minute or two, her mind went blank. In fact, I had a hard time seeing what she did for work, it was such a blur. I saw some antibody-associated problem with her thyroid. I saw that she might experience pressure in her chest. Was it hard for her to take a deep breath? At times, I saw nausea and an upset feeling in her stomach. Were there changes in estrogen and progesterone? I couldn't figure out if those hormonal changes made her crave carbohydrates, causing her to gain weight. I wondered if the weight gain led to problems with the joints in her lower body. In addition, I saw that there was something funny about her skin.

THE FACTS

Olivia complained of arthritis, psoriasis, thyroid problems, and panic attacks. However, her big problem was that she was failing at work. She was a legal assistant and couldn't keep up with the mountains of reading she had to do. It took her an entire weekend to write a report, a document that would take a colleague only a few hours to complete. She kept daydreaming, and her lack of focus was making her make mistakes. Olivia was perpetually behind the eight ball, frantically trying to keep up with her work so she wouldn't get fired. The panic and stress of trying to keep up with all that reading and writing was registering in her body in the form of arthritis, psoriasis, panic, and thyroid problems.

Olivia wanted to be a lawyer, but she was having trouble passing her LSATs. She would study for hours and hours and hours on exam booklets and sample tests, but then she would get caught in the quagmire of details. She confirmed, "That's me. Detail. Detail. I have all these charts, all these markers, all these files. I spend hours on homework, but no matter how long I'd spent on the papers, the professor said they were filled with grammatical errors and spelling errors, and I always missed the point of the assignment."

Olivia had taken the LSAT exam for law school three times and failed every single time. She had recently had a neuropsychological assessment and had been diagnosed with dyslexia as well as ADHD.

The Solution

Have you had trouble keeping up with the reading and writing in school and later at work? Have you been "laid off" or even fired from a job or lost promotions because of mistakes? Do you find yourself getting distracted by the problems of people around you?

You may have a language-based learning disability that makes your brain poorly adapted for a career that involves a lot of reading and writing. But your problem with left brain language disorder may leave you with an exaggerated intuitive ability that can help you in a healing or intuitive career. But beware: if you do want to use that emotional intuitive gift that your brain has as a byproduct of your language-based learning disability, you're still going to need help. Reading and writing are requirements for every career. Yes, they are, whether you like it or not. You're going to have to figure out how to hire or surround yourself with people who are "prosthetic" left brain types so that papers can be filed, insurance claim forms can be sent, and so on. Otherwise you'll find that you may be avoiding these most unpleasant, difficult details of business, not reading whole e-mails, not reading the details of contracts, and so on. Over time, needless to say, you'll find yourself in business and career hot water.

If you have dyslexia or mild language problems, you may also have an excessively emotional and intuitive brain that can lead you to have more "stress"-related health problems. Why? Many intuitives are very porous and very sensitive. They end up having a lot of autoimmune problems, joint problems, and ultimately their health can cause them to have trouble holding a regular job in the world. The work of Norman Geschwind indicates that people with dyslexia are more likely to have autoimmune illnesses, such as psoriatic arthritis, Hashimoto's disease, scoliosis, migraine headaches, and seizure disorders, to name only a few. Why is this so? It may be that when the brain is developing in the first trimester, if the left brain language areas are developing aberrantly, the thymus, the immune system area, is as well. This is called the Geschwind-Behan-Galaburda hypothesis, and it's very controversial. Every 10 years, a different study is published to support or refute it. If you have dyslexia—a left brain learning disorder with problems with language—though you might have a hyperintuitive right brain, the downside? You may have to deal with a variety of hard-to-treat health problems.

If this is you—if you have dyslexia, yet are porous and intuitive—fear not. You can capture your emotional intuitive gifts, but also capitalize on what language you do have in your brain. But you must shore up your immune system, because your intuitive gifts may lead to immune system problems. First, if you have problems with attention, go to the previous case in this chapter's clinic and find solutions to hone the focus in your brain, because attention and dyslexia tend to be brain styles that "travel together." Go to an acupuncturist and herbalist and have them help strengthen your immune system. If you have autoimmune illnesses, have them build up your kidney and liver yin. If you're concerned that you may have dyslexia, get a neuropsychological assessment for attention, learning, and memory. In addition to telling you if you have ADHD or dyslexia, the board-certified neuropsychologist will help you find a language-based learning center. These reading specialists use a multisensory way of teaching you how to read. By learning how to use multiple areas in your brain to read, you can work your way around any little aberrant spots of brain development.

Don't limit. Expand your education. Go to your nearest university and look for resources for individuals with dyslexia. Take classes. And if you do have a diagnosis of dyslexia, ask to have your exams given to you with extended times. Many individuals with dyslexia and ADHD get this kind of accommodation because in that format they are more able to demonstrate their grasp of the information. In addition, I would go to the career office at the university and talk about various career options that are suitable for your unique brain style. Naturally, if you have a language-based learning disability or dyslexia, you might not want to get a Ph.D. in English literature, because, as in this case, you'd have trouble keeping up with the reading and always be behind the eight ball, despite help from a reading specialist. By talking to your neuropsychologist or a career or vocational counselor at the university, you may be able to find out a vocation or career that is uniquely designed for your unique brain.

THE AFFIRMATIONS

Louise helps people understand that their different learning styles enable them to have the right career, one in which they'll be exceptional and gifted. Thus, all of us are disabled in one way or another if we're in the wrong career. In essence, Louise sees that the only learning disability any of us have is an inability to love our brain style. When we don't love our minds, we tend to have panic and anxiety, which over time may increase our tendency toward autoimmune problems. So Louise suggests a variety of affirmations. First, a total love and acceptance of our own identity, and second, an affirmation for the panic and anxiety we may experience when we are struggling to keep up in a career that's not adapted to our unique brain style, and then finally affirmations that address the health problems—perhaps, in the case of dyslexia, autoimmune problems—that may get worse when one is panicked or frustrated with one's learning style. Consider the following affirmations:

- For acceptance, the affirmation is "I am love. I now choose to love and approve of myself. I see others with love."

- For fear and anxiety affirmations, go to Chapter 2.

- For health problems like psoriasis, Hashimoto's disease, scoliosis, epilepsy, migraine headache, and others that you may have, go to Appendix B in the back of the book.

III. RIGHT BRAIN LEARNING DISORDERS

A right brain learning disorder is a developmental brain style in which you have difficulties in your day-to-day social and emotional awareness. The usual function of the right brain is being able to be aware of your feelings and simultaneously aware of someone else's. Akin to walking and chewing gum at the same time, we use our right brain to be aware of our nervousness and at the same time know that someone else near us is angry or sad. In addition to balancing our feelings and someone else's, the right brain helps us with boundaries—knowing where our feelings end and someone else's begin. In addition to handling, expressing, and comprehending emotion, the right brain also handles paying attention. Whether it's dividing attention between the radio and the road when you're driving, or your computer screen and what your boss is saying in the workplace, this is another juggling act that the right brain performs. Finally, our right hemisphere creates a three-dimensional map of our world. Whether it's being able to actually *read* a map, comprehend geometry, parallel park, or perceive distance and speed while driving, this visual-spatial aspect, though hard to explain, is obvious when you don't have it.

So, knowing the usual functions of the right brain, it may be easier for you to imagine what it's like to have been born with a unique right brain style:

- You may have difficulty with eye contact. Why? It may be difficult for you to handle your own feelings and balance those with awareness of emotions in someone else's face.

- You may have more difficulty expressing your feelings in words, and you may have an even harder time "reading" the expression of emotion inherent in someone else's facial expression or tone of voice.

- Social nuance may elude you. As you proceed through middle school and high school and beyond, you may feel like you're "on the outside looking in" socially. Other people may seem to be speaking a "social language" that you don't know. It's not quite shyness that you feel, it's more the awkwardness of not knowing what to say or do. Other people seem to just "know" the rules of engagement when it comes to dating, going to dances, schmoozing after work or on the job.

- Though you feel comfortable hanging out with a family member or a local historian or scientist or older teacher, when it comes to being around groups of people your own age, you feel uncomfortable. Some people have said you may have social anxiety. And then when you leave to go to college, it may be particularly difficult for you to share a room with a dorm-mate. You may find yourself arguing over details that are extremely important to you but that your roommate thinks are ridiculous.

- You tend to be detail-oriented, somewhat compulsive, and perfectionistic. Once you put something in its place, if someone moves it, you get anxious. You tend to be set in your routines.

- You tend to be better in such detail-oriented left brain fields as computers, engineering, and technology, but not social work, psychology, or anthropology. You have a hard time handling the political machinations that are required at work to move up in your career, and you don't understand why. If your work is executed flawlessly, why aren't you advancing as much as that smooth-talking, socially and politically skilled colleague who's not nearly as bright as you? You find yourself saying, "It's just not fair."

- You may feel closer to nature and prefer it to having someone nurture you. You may feel more entertained putting together models or Legos or working on a computer than sitting in a coffeehouse for hours talking to a friend.

- You're more likely to have allergies, especially digestive allergies to wheat. You're more likely to have muscle tightness and stiffness in your body, as well as insomnia. Alcoholism may run in your family. And if you are in a relationship, it's quite possible that your partner has tried to bring you into therapy to get you to talk about your feelings more. You've tried it, and, you know what, it wasn't the most productive or practical experience.

If this is you or a loved one, congratulations! Though your strengths may not be in your right brain functioning, nonetheless your left brain capacity for logic, details, and rational thinking in the areas of engineering, science, and math, or other areas that require a left brain thinking style, may be awe-inspiring. In essence, you may have the opposite of the brain style we looked at in the previous section, dyslexia. If dyslexia is a left brain learning disorder, an individual who has exaggerated right brain emotional and intuitive gifts, you are someone with a right brain learning disorder, someone with exaggerated left brain language, logic, and linear abilities. Often enough, people with these two opposite brain styles marry, and I've been known to say, tongue in cheek, that between the two of them they have a "complete brain." We tend to marry the part of the brain we don't have, or at least the part that doesn't function as well as the rest. This is perhaps what they mean when they say that opposites attract. So next time you look at your partner and want to change him or her, stop. Think about it. Is that really what you want to do? Because maybe, just maybe, between the two of you, you complement each other and help each other heal your minds so you can create wholeness.

However, if you've had a struggle with obvious or even subtle right brain symptoms, whether it's in groups of people, in relationships or finances, or at work, you can use medicines, nutritional supplements, affirmations, and intuition to create wholeness whether you're alone or in a relationship. Read on to the following story as we show you how.

PATRICK: THE PATHOLOGY OF SUPERIORITY

Patrick, age 39, called me because he was concerned about his health.

THE INTUITIVE READING

When I first read Patrick, I saw that he was very sensitive, especially in public places. I saw that it was hard for him to feel comfortable around people. Whether at work or at school, it felt like Patrick was only comfortable with people in the family he grew up with. On the other hand, I saw that Patrick was very comfortable with numbers and details, whether it was because they were tidy or because they were logical, it didn't matter. Was it that people made him uncomfortable? Intuitively, I couldn't see people around him, and I didn't see a partner or kids. Just Patrick alone in a room.

The Body

The first thing I noticed was that Patrick had very sensitive skin. It felt like red dots appeared on his skin, especially when he ate certain foods. He felt more or less healthy, with the exception of lifelong digestive allergies, specifically to wheat or some other food. These weren't those garden-variety wheat allergies that everyone is talking about these days. Patrick never could eat wheat since he was born. If he did, he would double over in pain.

The Facts

Patrick said he had gone from doctor to doctor, dermatologist to dermatologist, to deal with his eczema. No one could find out what he was allergic to, except wheat. In fact, ever since he was a child, he could neither eat wheat nor drink milk.

Patrick had called me not mainly for his physical health but for problems at work. He had gotten fired, not for the first time. He said, "I don't know what's wrong with these managers these days. They certainly aren't interested in doing things the right way." Patrick had worked as an administrative assistant in a publishing house, and then most recently at a line editing job, until he got fired once again, and now he was simply doing clerical work. It was an argument with an author over the difference between the words *that* and *which* that had caused the recent firing. Patrick told me, "A fact is a fact. I don't understand why people get so offended when you instruct them on the proper use of grammar and syntax."

It was clear that Patrick was having difficulty balancing his superb left brain language and logical skills with an understanding of right brain social and emotional nuance and politics. And he was unable to handle two opposing points of view, to balance his logical opinion with the opinions of people he worked with (including his superiors), believing that fact and logic trumped opinions, feelings, and positions. The imbalance led Patrick to perpetual frustration, depression, and anxiety. First he was angry, thinking *I'm right, they're wrong, things should be different*; then he was depressed because his unique intellectual abilities weren't valued; then he was anxious when he realized he'd lost his job and didn't know how he was going to pay his bills.

Patrick had no idea how to even express his frustration, depression, and anxiety, let alone understand why his boss fired him or was angry in the first place. However, the cumulative backlog of feelings got shunted to his adrenal gland, increasing his chance of releasing the stress hormone cortisol. Cortisol in turn increased his chance toward having worsening allergies in his body. Patrick added, "Oh, you'd be interested in this. I was in special education when I was a child because I talked late, but look at me now! I'm a very advanced English scholar, with a master's degree in English literature. Humph! So much for Special Ed!"

THE PATHOLOGY OF SUPERIORITY

Every single one of us has a genius. Like Patrick, you too may have an amazing ability that is somehow related to a weakness somewhere else in your brain. Like a coin with heads and tails, all of our brains have some area of a "deficiency" that is somehow matched with a superlative, of course, depending on degree. In its most extreme form, someone with a dramatic problem in their right brain may be labeled autistic and their superior abilities may earn them the label of an autistic savant. If you're someone with extreme weaknesses in your right brain, you needn't be autistic, I might add. Having extreme difficulty with social and emotional skills may biologically predispose you to having an exaggerated capacity for details, logic, science, and technology. You may be incredibly gifted at calculating numbers, performing technical feats with computer coding, or comprehending and replicating symphonies or art. However, your inability to work in a team environment or social setting will unveil your right brain emotional weaknesses. None of us are perfect. All of us have gradations of weakness to some degree in one hemisphere over the other. Some of us may be pseudo-savants in right brain emotional and intuitive capabilities that incline us toward being therapists, social workers, psychologists, creative artists, and so on. So what's the solution if you have an extreme brain style, whether it's the one in this section (extreme left brain skills and right brain deficiency) or the one we saw in the previous section (extreme right brain skills and a relatively weak left brain)?

The Solution

Notice we're getting away from diagnostic labels like dyslexia and right brain learning disability. You needn't have a diagnosis of extreme deficiency in either your right or your left brain to be able to utilize the solutions in this section or the one before. We all can learn how to identify weaknesses in one of our hemispheres versus the other and try to improve them so we can create wholeness in our minds. By utilizing both our right and our left brain to the best of our ability, we are in essence learning how to better use our whole brain, not just rest on the laurels of the side we're most comfortable with.

The first solution is to apply that dialectical principle of opposites from dialectical behavioral therapy—that is, that you can love yourself, your current brain style, just the way you are and paradoxically want to be even better. By improving the skills of your other hemisphere, you will not be "losing" your unique identity. You won't be becoming any less yourself. No one will think you're becoming "boring" or losing your individuality—that which makes you quirky or unusual, or stand out, or even excel. Loving yourself just the way you are *and* wanting to acquire skills in the hemisphere where you're weaker simply makes you adapt better in the world, and by using your whole mind to adapt to the world you'll be better able to communicate your unique genius and individuality.

The next solution is to augment your environment with people or tools to buff up that side of the brain that's not as strong. If you have extreme right brain skills, as in the previous section, you're going to need to hire—or marry—someone with left brain skills to help you negotiate the world of paperwork, documentation, and the standardized testing that is often required for getting one's credentials. Alternately, as in this section, if you tend toward left brain skills, with high abilities for order, perfection, logic, and technical capabilities—you need to supplement yourself with the opposite hemisphere as well. With extreme left brain logical capabilities, you may find yourself faltering when it's necessary to negotiate social nuance in the academic world to acquire tenure or in a career to deal with politics and schmoozing to work your way up through the ranks. In that sense, you need to marry, or hire, a right-brain-skilled individual who can coach you on how to say the right thing to the right person at the right time. Otherwise, your often logical, fact-based left-brain-focused mind may tend to step on the toes of those in your family and your work, offending and putting off people in a way you may not even be aware of.

The third solution is dialectical behavioral therapy or cognitive behavioral therapy. Using DBT or CBT may help you rewire and strengthen the brain pathways necessary to function with both brains in the world. Specifically, in DBT, one skill based on Tibetan Buddhism and mindfulness, called Wise Mind, is used to create a whole, balanced brain by helping you identify right brain emotional mind and balance its effects with left brain mental mind. This DBT skill helps you use mindfulness to observe, describe, and allow the creation of a gentle balance between both hemispheres in perception, thoughts, and ultimately how you act with friends, family, and colleagues in the world. There are many other techniques as well. However, a word of caution: if you think because you have done DBT or CBT for a period of six months, or a year, or more, now you're all set—your brain is normalized—think again! People who are born left-handed can teach themselves to be ambidextrous, using both hands—or hemispheres, I might add—to move about the world. But in their brain, they are always left-handed, and in times of stress or exhaustion or taxing life events, they will revert to their original, pure, inborn mind-set. Similarly, whatever therapies you do to help bolster or strengthen the hemisphere that's weaker will do the same: create a pseudo-ambidextrous ability in the brain. You can, to some degree, with effort and intention, have more of a whole brain and act accordingly in the world. However, during times of stress, anxiety, depression, grief, illness, you're going to need support from people or your environment to support the part of the brain that you're not naturally gifted in.

THE AFFIRMATIONS

Ultimately, whatever hemisphere you have weakness in, you may have had challenges with finances, work, and success as a result, struggling to "wrap your mind around" the task at hand. Whether it's the enormous amount of reading, writing, and details (for left brain learning problems) or the social and emotional challenges of managing bosses, committees, meetings, shifting alliances and emotional innuendo in families and at work may leave you with financial and career catastrophes that will bruise your self-esteem and self-image. Many of the affirmations that you'll want to use will involve addressing the problems you've had in your life with money, relationships, and work. Consider the following thought patterns that you may have and the corresponding affirmations from Louise:

- If you think no one appreciates you at work: "My work is recognized by everyone."

- If you always get dead-end jobs: "I turn every experience into an opportunity."

- If your boss is abusive: "I respect myself and so do others."

- If everyone expects too much of you: "I am in the perfect place and I am safe at all times."

- If your co-workers drive you crazy: "I see the best in everyone and help them bring out their most joyous qualities."

- If your job offers no creativity: "My thoughts are creative."

- If you think you'll never be successful: "Everything I touch is a success."

- If you believe there is no chance for advancement: "New jobs are opening all the time."

- If your job doesn't pay well: "I am open and receptive to new avenues of income."

- If your job is too stressful: "I am always relaxed at work."

- The general affirmation is "I give myself permission to be creatively fulfilled."

IV. Personality Styles—Finding Yourself

We spend our whole lives trying to find happiness, looking for it in families, relationships, money, work, children, activism in the world, education, and spirituality. But still we may not feel joy. You may not know it, but you've spent your whole life trying to learn how to be happy. You've been trying to mold your brain circuits toward peace. The Hebrew word *shalom* means "peace," but it also means "whole." And when we get older and perhaps wiser, we begin to look for peace and harmony between ourselves, others, and mankind in general. Think of it: in many a beauty pageant, when the participants are asked what their platform is, they say, "World peace." Whether that's true or said to evoke emotion in the viewer, happiness and peace seem to be that elusive essence that all of us are looking for. We spend our whole lives trying to learn how to acquire it.

Every single one of us is born with some difficulty, some challenge, in acquiring happiness and peace. Whether it's a problem with depression or irritability (Chapter 1), anxiety (Chapter 2), addiction (Chapter 3), learning (this chapter), and so on, not to mention health problems, we all try to file off the rough edges of our personality and shape ourselves so that we can come closer to peace. All of us have some weakness in our brain, some pattern of flaws in mood, anxiety, addiction, learning, and so on, that we need to unravel so we can better adapt to the world. This pursuit of happiness is, in essence, learning how to shape our personality.

This section is devoted to the disorder that all of us have in our psyche—the part of our personality, wired in our brain, that we spend our entire life working on or working through to create happiness. In essence, when we are healing our mind with medicine, affirmations, and intuition, the wholeness—the peace—we are trying to achieve is what we call "finding ourselves." Finding yourself is trying to add those little bits and pieces to your psyche that are weak or missing that make it harder for the nutritional supplements, medicines, or therapies of any kind to fix your depression, irritability, anxiety, or other brain problems in a lasting way.

So how is personality wired in the brain? Personality is a product of temporal lobe emotions and frontal lobe capacity to curb your feelings so you can keep that job or relationship or fit into society. More or less, there is a continuum of personality styles between three basic categories. Mind you, do not think I am saying you are one or the other—it's a continuum! At one extreme, there are people who are more hyper-temporal-lobe, that is, less emotionally restrained. The other extreme is more hyper-frontal-lobe, people who have more of the brakes on and are more restrained. The third style is a combination of characteristics in the temporal lobe and the frontal lobe creating uniqueness, distinctive personalities, and eccentricities that often make a person feel like a black sheep or an outsider looking in. Because they swing between the first two personality styles, at times they are prone to emotional intensity and at other times they can be extremely anxious, restrained, and aloof.

To create wholeness in the brain, one needs balance. Yin needs yang; we need to offset our right brain with our left; and when it comes to personality, we need to balance our frontal lobe and temporal lobe. Just as in the last two sections, where one hemisphere is stronger than the other, if your temporal lobe or frontal lobe dominates over the other, you may find it's harder for you to get closer to happiness and peace. Your depression, anxiety, or irritability, the learning disabilities and addictions you have, not to mention the issues with memory, intuition, and spirituality (which you'll read about in the upcoming chapters), may afford you both challenges and gifts. To create wholeness, in this learning styles section, again we learn to love ourselves just the way we are *and* want to be better.

It's easy enough to understand that a weaker frontal lobe will make you less restrained and a stronger frontal lobe will make you more restrained. But what about those people who are eccentric and unique? What do they do—do they have to rework both brain areas? Many individuals with this unique, eccentric brain style may feel safer with spirit and the divine than they do with people on earth. In essence, these individuals' primary relationships and work are with spirit. People with this brain style may be mystics or monks or work in spiritual fields, and often may have difficulty feeling accepted by family or society in general. If you are one of these people—and from time to time I may include myself in this category—you may often want to say, "I love myself, so why do I need to fit in in the world?" Often the things people are concerned about in today's society seem superficial, irrelevant, and, to use a word that my dear friend and colleague Caroline Myss uses, pedestrian. Well, if you have this brain style in which you feel safer with spirit than with people on earth, too bad. You are still living on the earth. And as long as you do walk on the earth, you too are a pedestrian! Often people with this brain style have a variety of complex, hard-to-treat health problems, including neurological disorders like migraine headaches and seizures, learning disorders of many kinds, thyroid problems, cancers, weight and blood sugar issues, digestive allergies, chronic immune system problems, and multiple joint and spinal issues. Many of the great saints, I might add, who were not what you'd call run-of-the-mill citizens, were unique and eccentric and had both unrestrained personalities at times (hypo-frontal-lobe) and at other times overly restrained. More on this in Chapter 6.

If this is you, though you may think you're comfortable in this brain style, hanging out with spirit, away from earthbound citizens, think again. Your health is likely to suffer if you don't walk with the rest of the herd on earth. You may notice that you and those great saints have something in common: a lot of health problems. All people's health is improved by having a social network, so if you are in the third category, and specifically a unique person set apart by the quality of spirituality—a monk of sorts— find yourself a bunch of other monks and mystics to hang out with. It will improve your mood, anxiety, irritability, thyroid and hormonal issues, immune system and weight problems, to name only a few mind-body challenges.

Look among these three styles. You may find you're not as extreme at one time of your life as at another. This section on learning styles is about how to shape your personality so you can get along better in the world, whether it's in your family, in your relationships, in your work, with money, and so on. So when you go through those three basic types on the continuum of personality styles, ask yourself, did you feel that you had difficulty fitting in in grade school, in high school, in college, and at a job? Do you have difficulty curbing your frustration when you have to deal with other people's expectations? Is it hard for you to go after what you want if you're especially aware that you may hurt someone else's feelings or even make them angry? These kinds of questions that prompt your unique brain style—they're endless! But they illuminate your personality style, that is, how you deal with the delicate balance between your feelings and someone else's, between what you want and what society as a whole wants.

We spend our whole lives filing the rough edges off of our frontal lobe and temporal lobe personality so we can modify our answers to these questions. After working with medicines, supplements, therapies, and affirmations, it may be easier to utilize the circuits in our brain between our frontal lobe and temporal lobe to feel like we "fit in" just a little bit more. And after using all those solutions, we may have just a little bit of an easier time curbing our frustration when a boss, mate, child, or parent is bearing down with demands. And after healing our minds throughout our lives with medicines, supplements, therapy, and affirmations, it may be just a little bit easier for us to go after what we want, even if we're aware that someone we care about may get angry. By learning across your lifetime with all the solutions in this section, which shape your personality circuits between your temporal lobe and your frontal lobe, you'll be better able to juggle your feelings with someone else's and what you want with what society wants. And in Chapter 6, you will learn how to use your right brain and left brain, frontal lobe and temporal lobe, to begin the process of balancing your feelings and what you want with your soul and the divine.

WHY ARE THEY LIKE THAT?

From time to time, I do readings for people who have a difficult mother, a difficult father, a difficult child, and so on. They say things like: "We can't get along. He's so moody. She's so irritable. They stole from me. They abused me. They've been in and out of rehab. They've been in and out of jail. Why are they like that? Why are they so difficult? Why? Why? Why? If they could only act normally, life would be better. If they could only change, my health would be better. If they could only treat me better, life would be sublime." If, if, if.

Here's the best way I can explain it: someone with an extreme developmental disorder that causes difficulty with these frontal lobe/temporal lobe connections is similar to someone who has, say, a developmental disorder at birth. Some "handicaps" are more obvious than others. For example, some children are born with a motor disorder called cerebral palsy. When they start walking, you can see that they lack fluid, smooth movement. So it's obvious when they start walking—you see the flaw in their frontal lobe movement areas. Their "handicap" is very visible earlier in their life because those brain areas develop early. However, the frontal lobe circuits to curb moodiness, irritability, follow rules in society, and so on—those circuits don't develop until your teens and 20s. So if a person has a developmental disorder in those brain circuits, the "handicap" is less obvious, because it doesn't involve walking or talking. Those biological flaws in the brain cause developmental effects that are in the personality, which can be profoundly handicapping, as only someone who is a parent, significant other, family member, or spouse can attest.

Someone with cerebral palsy or a speech problem will be able to comprehend their flaw and use the appropriate medicines, nutritional supplements, therapies, and affirmations to help themselves. However, unfortunate as it is, individuals who have extreme frontal lobe deficits in judgment, social restraint, and rules don't have that insight or the desire to shape their personality in healthier directions. They are very satisfied with the way they are and painfully believe that all their problems, be they legal, financial, vocational, or otherwise, are the fault of people around them. And so when I work with someone who says their mother was selfish or "narcissistic," or their father was a sociopath and was in jail, or their child broke into houses and got arrested several times, I try to explain this extreme frontal lobe/temporal lobe developmental brain disorder to them. Although it does not make these individuals less responsible for their behavior, it's important that we understand they were born with brains that challenge them.[13]

It's with this understanding of personality types, personality quirks, and shaping one's personality toward happiness that we go on to the following case.

SARAH: ESCAPING PERPETUAL CRISIS

Sarah called me for a reading because she said she was having trouble getting to sleep.

THE INTUITIVE READING

When I first started reading Sarah, her house felt like a M.A.S.H. unit. I could hear the phones going around and around and around, ringing, ringing, ringing. Her thoughts would go around and around in her head. I had a hard time seeing Sarah in a significant relationship with anybody else other than her phone. Sarah seemed to work long hours into the night at some kind of job; it seemed like she was always paying bills, paying bills, paying bills. And then I would see Sarah on the phone trying to get through to someone, trying to change his or her point of view.

THE BODY

There was pressure on Sarah's head. It felt like she was hitting her head against a brick wall. Did she have problems with antibodies directed against her thyroid? I saw a change in heart rhythm, some kind of skipping of a beat. I wondered if Sarah was concerned about densities in her chest region around her breasts, especially on the left side. In addition, I wondered whether Sarah's frustration and panic increased her adrenal gland's capacity to make estrogen and cortisol. However, as I was reading her body, I kept seeing her on the phone trying to get through to someone.

THE FACTS

Sarah told me that, yes, she had been diagnosed with breast cancer in her left breast, but she told me the reading was really about her daughter, Ruby. She said, "You're right. I was always on the phone trying to get through to my daughter. My daughter has had a very painful life. She's been struggling with unstable mood and behavior throughout her whole life. Although she's doing better since we've paid for her to go to all these expensive rehabs for alcohol abuse and cocaine, we're just not able to get the medicines stable for her depression and panic." Sarah didn't know if her daughter had a personality disorder, PTSD, or bipolar II.

THE SOLUTION

Are you, like Sarah, thinking your problem in your mind and body is only one symptom? Sarah first thought her central problem was insomnia. Then, after a while, she admitted she was worried about her daughter, whom she couldn't get through to, because her daughter might have some personality disorder.

All of our personalities affect our moods, our anxiety, and our capacity to learn, whether it's in its most severe form, as in Sarah's daughter, or in its mildest form, or somewhere in between. If you yourself have a problem with depression, irritability, panic, addiction, or an array of health problems, don't just work on each of these individual problems. Learn to shape the features of your personality so you can better adapt between your feelings and someone else's and society in general. Otherwise, you may find that medicines, nutritional supplements, therapies, and affirmations will work for only a while. And then invariably something will change in your family or relationship, your finances, or your work, and then you're likely to lose it. Lose the balance of wholeness you'd achieved. You'll think you need to tinker with the meds or the supplements, switch therapists, add affirmations, or look for food or environmental allergies and so on. You may even for the moment consider a variety of relationship allergies as well, thinking that removing a person or a job, or even moving geographically, will make you happier. Maybe, but you know the phrase: "Wherever you go, there you are."

Everyone has someone in their life like Sarah's daughter. Everyone is going to find someone, whether it's a mother or a father, a boyfriend or girlfriend or boss, that they'll feel the impulse to "get through to." If only we could get them to change, we would be happier, and then we would be not depressed, not anxious, definitely not irritable, and we would sleep better, eat better, and be at peace. World peace. I don't think so! It doesn't work that way. If your health and happiness are dependent on someone else changing, you have problems.

Cognitive behavioral therapy, dialectical behavioral therapy, mindfulness, and affirmations are all tools that can help you learn to change someone—and that someone is you. Yes, you may suggest for a minor child whose moods and behavior are veering out of control to get into the right kind of therapy or medicine. All the while, though, we all need to learn that when someone in our life has mind-body challenges, we may help them but we also need to employ a DBT skill called Radical Acceptance. Radical Acceptance involves learning the balance between willfulness—changing a situation—and willingness to accept that things will happen the way they happen.[14] Radical Acceptance does not mean that you are pleased with the results of what's happened to your friend, family member, and so on, or that you feel it's fair, right, or just. Radically accepting the situation in your life that's "keeping you up at night" is the only way out of your suffering. To perpetually try to "get through to them," to "change them," only increases your chance of being chronically depressed, irritable, and anxious, and such emotions may potentially lead you to addiction and a host of health problems. We know that those chronic emotions can injure your adrenal gland hormones, changing levels of estrogen and cortisol, influencing your immune system.

I suggest you seek out dialectical behavioral therapy. Go to www.behavioraltherapy.org and ask for someone who knows DBT. When you call, they may or may not ask you if you have borderline personality disorder. However, DBT is also often used for many people with medication-resistant depression, anxiety, moodiness, and PTSD, as well as family members of people with severe disorders of mental illness. If you are in a long-term relationship with someone who has these kinds of emotional problems, understand that the perpetual crisis will increase your own chance of perpetual health problems. DBT and CBT will help you figure out more skillful ways of creating peace and wholeness in your life rather than simply "changing them."

THE AFFIRMATIONS

If you want to create wholeness and happiness in your life, join the club. We're all in it. You can learn how to love yourself just the way you are and also unveil and unearth more and more of your true self through affirmations. Consider the following affirmations to help you heal your mind to create wholeness and happiness:

- I am willing to change.
- Life is very simple.

- Remember we are dealing with thoughts, and thoughts can be changed.

- We can change our attitude toward the past.

- In my mind I have total freedom.

- I now move into a new space of consciousness where I am willing to see myself differently. I am willing to create new thoughts about myself and my life. My new thinking becomes my new experiences.

- The universe is more than willing to manifest my new beliefs, and I accept this abundant life with joy, pleasure, and gratitude, for I am deserving. I accept it. I know it to be true.

Chapter 5

MEMORY

Now that you've read this far in the book, we take all of the information you've read and we turn to the subject of memory. What is memory? Memory is taking what we've experienced in the past and turning it into wisdom. You can read all kinds of esoteric academic books about what memory is or isn't, how to sharpen it, or what happens when you lose it. However, if we can't incorporate those two common themes about what memory is, we will not be able to help ourselves when this important brain function seems to slip beyond our grasp.

Before we talk about being worried about losing our memory, now or in the future, it's important to understand how living in the present impacts the memory circuits in our brain and body. Vis-à-vis how our memory works, connecting the times in our life, I watched the movie *Alice through the Looking Glass*, where Alice tries to connect the past, present, and future. But the Mad Hatter, who is allegedly not supposed to have that much wisdom, shows he actually does when he states, profoundly, "Don't try to connect the past and future, because it will blow up the present." Actually, I hope I'm remembering that quote correctly! In fact, that's the point: to some degree, all of us have quirky memory, whether it's due to a tendency in our brain toward depression, anxiety, irritability, learning problems like ADHD, dyslexia, right brain disorder, or others. Whether you've had trauma across your life, physical and emotional health problems in the past or the present, all these issues can distort your memory circuitry to a degree. How you laid down memory in your brain in the past and the wisdom you receive in the future really depend on how you heal your mind to create wholeness in the present. Maybe it's true: to biologically or psychologically try to alter your memory in the past, if it takes so much time in your present life, you simply won't be living, acquiring and learning knowledge for the future.

So therefore, as we learn about memory and all its disorders, and you're afraid of losing it, whether you feel that your brain isn't working well now or you're afraid of getting Alzheimer's disease in the future, stop. Yes, it's important to work on one's brain and body to maximize one's health now and in one's later years, with nutritional supplements, herbs, medicines, cognitive behavioral therapies, affirmations, and so on. But the most potent medicine that will dementia-proof your brain now and for the rest of your life is daily learning, changing, and acquiring wisdom as an individual and alongside everyone else in your world.

It is possible to live throughout our lives with a keen, sharp mind. We are not destined to have dementia. I repeat: we are not destined to have dementia or other forms of memory loss. I remember when I was 12, we would hear that this person had hardening of the arteries or that person had "senility" (another word for dementia). At that point, it seemed that losing one's "mind" was the inevitable consequence of growing older. I'm telling you now it's not. In the 21st century, we see that many parts of our memory as we get older actually are sharper than when we were younger.

Yes, you are noticing that your memory works differently as you age. It's supposed to. As you get older, you have more experience laid down in all the networks of your brain. Perhaps it takes more time to come up with that name or that term or that word. Is it because your mind has to work its way through all that wisdom that's accumulated in the libraries of your mind? Amid all the stacks of accumulated knowledge you've acquired, it's no wonder that in normal aging our mind is supposed to act more slowly and be less impulsive. Understand that you do not want the mind of a 20-year-old, or a teenager even, who by definition has several decades less of accumulated information and experience to rifle through when it comes to retrieving a name or date or incident. Be kind with yourself. Understand your library of memory in your mind is much thicker than theirs. Have some respect for how the magnificent instrument of memory matures in a healthy aging brain. We're going to help you love and appreciate your memory, whatever age you are, and whatever has happened in your life.

WAYS OF LOOKING AT MEMORY

Memory is an important part of our intuition—it lets us know when our mind may be "elsewhere," empathically or virtually keying in to some other form of consciousness. Whether it's the pain of a loved one or a need to focus on some other task or concern, your memory and attention may seemingly veer off course when intuitively your mind has "a mind of its own," leading you to a source of information you wouldn't rationally have considered.

Memory also becomes a source for our intuition. How? Memory is laid down in the network of images and symbols and sensations in our brain and body. When our intuitive guidance speaks to us, giving us some key information about our life or the life of a loved one, our intuition may retrieve from those "memory banks" in our brain and body images, symbols, or sensations. Here's one example. If you witnessed an automobile accident in the past, you have a memory of it in your brain and body. The sights, the sounds, and the feeling of horror are like a 3-D movie that you carry around with you your whole life long without even being aware of it. Then, later on in life, perhaps, if you are about to create a serious commitment with someone who's very similar to an abusive partner in the past, you may actually have a terrifying dream of a car accident. The imagery, the loud crash, the sight of two cars colliding and almost totally destroying themselves may wake you up in a cold sweat, shaking with terror. Only when you tell a close confidant about your dream may they ask you, "What do you think about your relationship with so-and-so? Do you think you're going down that same path again? Do you think you're going to have another destructive relationship like you've had with your last three partners?" Your intuition, by way of the dream, uses memory of the past to warn you about the future consequences of your actions in the present.

How Memory Is Made

The key memory centers in the brain are like tollbooths on a highway. Information comes into your brain and goes either to the hippocampus or to the amygdala.[1]

Traumatic memory and body memory go through the amygdala. Less emotionally charged memory goes through the hippocampus. Alzheimer's disease initially affects the hippocampus, but then, like a brush fire, spreads to other select areas of the brain.

When something moves you emotionally, the sights, the sounds, the smells, the body sensations, all that information travels through the hippocampus and then, like a network, is stored throughout your brain. However, if a situation is especially traumatic, filled with terror and grief and even rage, memory is more likely to go through the amygdala and not the hippocampus. Whereas if memory is laid down through the hippocampus, you're more likely to be able to talk about in detail what you "remember," in the case of especially traumatic events, since the sights, the sounds, the smells, and the body feelings are diverted through the amygdala, you are less likely to be able to talk about them. Instead, your body tends to "talk" about it. How? When reverberations of the event spread through your brain and body, you don't really talk about them as much, but your body sure does through health problems, unhealthy habits and relationships, and poor choices. If we have long-term pain and suffering, whether it's in our family, at school, at work, or around us, as in war, the high levels of stress hormones—epinephrine and cortisol—make it hard for the hippocampus to lay down memory so we can talk about the event in detail and process and release it.

Traumatic memory has specific implications when we consider the field of medical intuition, health, and disease. If you have had a particularly painful past in your family (first center), relationships or finances (second center), physical, emotional, or sexual abuse (third center), parental neglect and abandonment (fourth center), and so on, these regions of your body, emotional centers, may let you know later on in life when you are in a situation that seems similar or even identical to your past trauma. Immune system disorders, joint pain, skin disorders (first center), reproductive, hormonal, chronic lower back or hip pain, bladder problems (second center), eating disorders, obesity, addiction (third center), chronic depression, panic, asthma, palpitations, or breast disease (fourth center)—symptoms in these areas may be the only signal you get to warn you that your present is recreating your past trauma.

Using medical intuition, we can learn to access the memory that's laid down in our body. It's never too late to "work through," for a limited time, with a counselor, those traumas that have happened in the past so we can reframe and forgive them. Part of the wisdom that we accumulate in life is learning to love ourselves, mind, body, and soul, just the way we are. This is what Louise Hay teaches us. One important element of loving ourselves is appreciating and radically accepting how our brain and body have been wired for memory through what has happened to us in our past. If you have a history of trauma, you can maximize your hippocampal memory through nutritional supplements, herbs, medicines, affirmations, and cognitive behavioral therapy. You can also learn to use medical intuition to access memory as it is laid down and stored in your body through a network of health or disease. Both mind memory (hippocampus) and body memory (amygdala) are essential forms of our memory system. To denigrate one or the other is not just denigrating who you are, it's not healthy and it's not going to help you have better memory. You're going to learn in the All Is Well Clinic how your unique mind-body memory needs to be sharpened to create wholeness. But first, the recipe.[2]

CREATING A HEALTHY MEMORY SYSTEM WITH NUTRITIONAL SUPPLEMENTS, HERBS, MEDICINES, AND NEUROTRANSMITTERS

Want to maximize your memory? Want to sharpen your capacity to retain what you're reading or have rapid-fire recall? Whether you're taking nutritional supplements, herbs, or medicines to make you sharp, it's important to understand there are a variety of ways to approach brain-body memory health:

- Reduce inflammation.
- Protect your brain from injury.
- Stop reliving trauma from the past. Radically accept and forgive those who've traumatized you.
- Support your immune system.
- Exercise.
- Minimize smoking and drinking.
- Treat depression, anxiety, irritability, and addiction.
- Learn every day. Read, and expose yourself to ever-changing styles of music, art, culture, people, and language.
- Increase love and joy from multiple sources: people, children, animals, nature, and spirituality.
- Get support. Resist the need to always be alone.
- Accept change in your life, in the people around you, and in society as a whole.
- Provide your brain with the molecules it needs for memory, including acetylcholine, GABA,

serotonin, norepinephrine, dopamine, and possibly hormones as well.

Let's look at this in some more detail.

- When it comes to the brain and Alzheimer's disease, acetylcholine is the most important neurotransmitter for memory. So, as you age, you don't want to take medicines or supplements or over-the-counter drugs that get rid of acetylcholine. Such over-the-counter sleep pills or medicines that treat allergies get rid of acetylcholine and will make your brain feel like a Q-tip. So, Benadryl and other allergy medicines or sleep pills can make your brain fuzzy. Ask your physician or pharmacist to go through your med list to find out which medicines are "anticholinergic." Then get rid of them.

- Ask yourself, have you had several blows to your head and possibly injuries to your brain? Whether you've been a soccer player or a football player, been in multiple car accidents, you need to take special care of your brain circuits for memory. In addition, if your childhood home had a lot of physical violence, consider the following. Did someone in your family get hit in the head repeatedly? If you witnessed a parent or sibling receive this kind of abuse, whether you remember it or not, you may have been a recipient of similar treatment. If you have a problem with your memory and have been in any of these situations, whether it's sports, an accident, or violence, get a neuropsychological assessment for attention, learning, and memory to find out if the test can pick up signs of traumatic brain injury. Though controversial, for people with brain injury, acupuncture or hyperbaric oxygen treatment may be helpful. Both may increase cerebral blood flow, helping you either increase plasticity—a rewiring of brain pathways around your injury—or increase efficiency in the memory you actually have.

And learn, learn, learn, learn, learn! Brain injury gets better over time. And although there is a lot of literature about people with something called chronic traumatic encephalopathy, the neurodegenerative disorder that occurs in people who have had multiple concussions or brain injuries, that is, like in boxing or football, it's never too late to use nutritional supplements, herbs, or medicines to try to clean up brain injury. When using nutritional supplements, herbs, hyperbaric oxygen, or acupuncture to encourage plasticity, new blood vessels may form and perhaps this disorder can be circumvented.

But understand there are some things that can make your memory worse. Alcohol is notorious for compounding brain injuries over time. If you have anxiety, you may be especially likely to use alcohol and have a hard time stopping. (See Chapter 3.) Alcohol doesn't just further injure brain pathways that interconnect memory. It alters B6 and B12, vitamins that are important for serotonin metabolism. If you find that you're using alcohol to treat anxiety, depression, and anger, you really need to get help. Not only does alcohol mess up critical sleep that's important for memory, it also disrupts your memory centers that produce neurotransmitters over time.

- If you have a chronic immune system dysfunction like lupus, rheumatoid arthritis, chronic fatigue, fibromyalgia, Lyme, or exposure to environmental toxicities like lead, mercury, and others, you may at times feel like you are in brain fog or delirium. (See Chapter 1 for solutions on brain fog.) In addition to a disruption in mood, chronic immune problems can disrupt memory pathways via chronic inflammation.

Cytokines or other inflammatory mediators, as in the case of allergy, histamines, can make you feel as if your thoughts are like trying to wade through chocolate pudding. Consider eliminating wheat, dairy, or other foods that may aggravate your allergy, autoimmune problem, or chronic infection. These food intolerances, not necessarily allergies, may make your brain fog mood/attention/memory problem worse.

- Do you have problems with insomnia? Insomnia in itself can disrupt your memory in a profound way. Sleep makes your brain create the neurotransmitter acetylcholine. At night when you dream, when you go through REM, you have microseizures (see chapter 6), little events that produce the memory neurotransmitter acetylcholine. One of the best things you can do to improve your memory and improve your neurochemistry for memory is to get enough sleep, hopefully eight hours a night.

If you've had depression and irritability plus insomnia, consider some of the solutions in Chapter 1. If you've had anxiety, panic, and trauma plus problems getting to sleep and staying asleep, consider the solutions in Chapter 2. If you've tried everything, like 5-HTP, passion flower, lemon balm, melatonin, not to mention altering your environment by removing technology, manipulating shades, and so on, consider getting a sleep study at your nearby major medical center. Sometimes there are treatment programs that can be very effective in retraining your brain and body for regular, more restful and efficient sleep. Finally, as long as you haven't had a history of addiction to alcohol, Valium, or any other addictive substance, when it comes to memory and insomnia this is not a time for pride and stoicism. If all supplements, nutritional remedies, and other "natural" solutions have failed, medicine may be what you need to get to sleep. If it means using medicine to get enough acetylcholine to save your memory, it's worth it.[3]

MEMORY AND AFFIRMATIONS

Past trauma, through cortisol and epinephrine, can "gum up" or clog our precious memory circuitry. To literally dilute the impact of traumatic memory, thoughts, and images that are distributed throughout your brain and body, consider Louise Hay's mirror work. Think about it, you've actually been doing mirror work your whole life—just not mirror work that involves healthy affirmations. Whether it's due to painful family, relationship, financial, or work experiences in the past and the present, you may have found yourself looking in the mirror and consciously or unconsciously saying, *Growing older frightens me. People scare me. I'm afraid to be alone. I'll never be able to face old age. Gee, I look old! How long have I had those wrinkles? My skin looks so saggy. Why don't they love me? If only I weren't so fat. Who'd want to have sex with someone with these hips? I'm stuck in this job. Who's ever going to hire someone like me, since I'm so stupid?*

Louise Hay's mirror work involves looking at our mirror image so we can change how we see ourselves over time. You've been doing mirror work your whole life and you've been doing affirmations your whole life, but maybe they haven't been healthy. Perhaps while you're driving in the left lane, in a moment of exasperation, you've found yourself saying, "Why are these people so stupid?" only to find yourself looking in the mirror a few days later and saying to yourself, *Why am I so stupid? Why can't I figure this out?* You may have gone to the food court in the mall and seen someone with something of a weight problem wearing a T-shirt tucked into stretch pants, and mumbled under your breath, "I'd never wear anything like that. Don't they know what they look like?" only to later in the week, while you're getting ready to go out, look in the mirror, examine your outfit, and say to yourself, *I can't believe how fat I'm getting. No matter what I put on, I look so fat.* The affirmation you've uttered in the car and later in the food court, you've also done as mirror work at home.

These thoughts that you've uttered privately and/or in the mirror, like weeds, take over your brain and body in the form of memory networks. You can't remove them, really. People say they can do that through a variety of means; EMDR, and perhaps tapping, may have some mechanism for manipulating access to these traumatic memories. However, the only way you could remove them permanently would be to remove whole chunks of your brain matter (it has been done), not to mention parts of your body. There has to be another way.

You can dilute your bad memories with healthy affirmations. Saying over and over again in the mirror work, "I love myself just the way I am, I love myself just the way I am" competes with hearing "You are stupid, you are stupid." If you heard 3 times, "You are worthless!" and you say 100 times, "I love myself," you don't remove "You are worthless." You can't. It's in your brain. But now you have 100 more instances of hearing you're smart, and you learn to create relationships and settings now where you hear, "You're smart." And "You're so smart!" competes with "What an idiot you are," and after a while, the criticism has less of an effect, because you've diluted the unhealthy with healthy. For every 10 unhealthy affirmations and mirror work we've done in our life, we can perhaps attempt to do 20, 30, or even 40 healthier affirmations or mirror work to dilute the effects of the prior ones.

There are people who say they've erased traumatic memories. Well, I'm not going to say they didn't. However, there may be a functional reason why we all experience trauma. What? Trauma could actually have some positive effect in our lives? Not to excuse from responsibility those who injured us. But when we experience trauma, we get to overcome it and become something different, something stronger, more resilient, and may I say, somewhat wiser. Think Mahatma Gandhi. Nelson Mandela. Wilma Rudolph. Pick a cultural icon. Why do they become icons, anyway? Because they have transcended their painful past toward greatness. As a culture we create icons so we can see that we too are capable of greatness, that we also can transcend tragedy and trauma and in spite of it create an amazing, wise self. We don't want to forget who we were; we certainly don't want to hate who we are. *And* we want to be better.[4]

THE ALL IS WELL CLINIC

Just as with mood, anxiety, addiction, and learning disorders, there are many facets to memory. Therefore, there are many solutions. All of us have some concern of one kind or another with memory. Whether you've had problems with remembering in the past or present or you're concerned about your future, join me in the All Is Well Clinic, where you can learn the solutions to your unique memory concerns.

I. Depression's Long-Term Effect on Memory

Have you had an accumulation, a backlog, of grief in your life? Has depression been a perennial problem in your life? If so, long-term sadness, despair, loneliness, and unhappiness can chip away at the health of your brain's memory circuits. After decades of disappointment and sorrow with family, money, marriage, work, children, or even unrelenting catastrophic health problems, you may feel your memory is but a fog. Going from doctor to doctor, you may ask, "Is this really normal aging?" After tinkering with hormones, whether estrogen, DHEA, or cortisol for adrenal fatigue, not to mention a variety of nutritional supplements and herbs, you may still find that your mind and your memory are not what you'd like them to be. It may be that the slow drip of depression, the decades of anguish, rejection, melancholy, and sadness, have energetically and biochemically corrupted your memory circuits.

Consider the following feelings and thoughts. Do these sound like you?

THOUGHTS AND FEELINGS

- For lots of years over the past decades, I have been so sad and unhappy, but somehow I've managed to press on.

- Often I feel my future is hopeless; however, I try to look for mind-body solutions to create changes.

- As I look back on my past, whether it's family, finances, relationships, or work, I find myself feeling sad and wishing I could have figured out how to find happiness.

- Ever since I was very young, when someone around me is in pain or suffering, I usually feel guilty, sad, and distraught if I can't help them.

BODY/BEHAVIOR

- It's hard for me to remember when I've had long periods of excitement, optimism, and cheerfulness, no matter what I do to try to find happiness, whether it's being in nature, exercise, entertainment, movies, music, or friends.

- I cry easily. For most of my life I've spent a lot of time crying, and, I might add, not good tears.

- For much of my life I've easily gotten irritated by my environment, whether it's crowds, noises, intense light, or anything overstimulating.

- For a long time it's been hard for me to make decisions.

- For most of my life my body has felt weighted down with fatigue and exhaustion.

If you are someone who has fatigue, lethargy, and the mental and physical fatigue that goes along with lifelong sadness and depression, you may find that your mood is in part what is making your memory less sharp. There may be other elements that are causing you to have concerns about your memory. After you read the following case, read on to the other sections as well.

If many of these statements apply to you, you may have imbalances in your brain and body in dopamine, norepinephrine, serotonin, and other mood neurotransmitters. Please read Chapter 1 on mood and consider talking to a trained professional to get support to help you manage your moods so they don't become one preventable source of memory problems. Join me in the following case study so you can learn more solutions to help you manage moods and memory.

SUSAN: DO I HAVE ALZHEIMER'S DISEASE?

Susan, 57, called me because she was concerned about her memory.

THE INTUITIVE READING

When I looked at Susan's life, it seemed like she was running around, being everything to everybody. Was this because she was trying to escape this sense of sadness or grief sitting on her chest? It seemed like there had been a series of losses in her family. Had loved ones recently left her? It felt like Susan was running around, taking care of everybody else's needs in her family, cooking, cleaning, being a perennial mother.

THE BODY

I saw an overbearing pressure in Susan's head. Was this a tightness in her blood vessels? I looked at her neck, and once again, I saw that her blood vessels had difficulty maintaining stable pressure. Her body felt heavy, like it was weighted down. I saw problems with blood sugar regulation. In the past, were there problems with a buildup in her uterine wall? Did she have a surgery there? I sensed that at times Susan felt a pressure in her chest and it was hard to take a deep breath.

THE FACTS

Susan said that she was "big-boned," but no one would really think that she was overweight, even though the doctors said she was 50 pounds too heavy. Susan admitted she had a backlog of grief: she had lost her brother to cancer after taking care of her mother for over a decade with Alzheimer's disease. Years ago, Susan had had a hysterectomy for a fibroid after years of heavy bleeding and anemia, and she had taken steroids for asthma. Susan wanted to know if this was the cause of her memory problems. On the other hand, she asked, was she going to get the same memory problems as her mother, who had Alzheimer's? "No matter what I do, I can't balance my hormones nor fix my adrenal fatigue enough to make my mind clear."

THE SOLUTION

Have you had one person after another leave you? Have you had one loss after another? Sit down now and count the events that have left you grief-stricken.

- Family: how many people have died?
- Divorces, breakups, children moving away?
- How many financial catastrophes, bankruptcies, or legal problems?
- Job loss, layoff, or even retirement? Even though retirement may be a relief in that you don't have to work anymore, you still have a loss in your daily schedule, the daily exposure to people at work and in society.
- Life-threatening illnesses?

First you go to your doctor to find out if you're losing your memory, and they say, "It's just normal aging." If your memory problems occur around the setting of menopause, chances are this isn't due to Alzheimer's disease but to the biochemical changes in your brain that result from hormonal ups and downs. The area that lays down memories in your brain, the hippocampus, has estrogen and progesterone receptors. When estrogen goes up and down, your capacity to lay down memories via the hippocampus may go up and down. Thus, you may have problems with focus and attention, and you may feel that you are getting Alzheimer's disease. If you feel that you're just so confused, you may want to, in the short term, turn to bioidentical estrogen and progesterone to treat your cognitive symptoms. What's important to know is that your brain fog and memory problems are temporary. Memory symptoms at this time are not about the level of estrogen in your saliva or blood, so if you keep checking those levels, understand that memory problems are due to the changing levels of estrogen that cause memory symptoms at this time. When the hormone levels stabilize after five or ten years, you will reach a new steady state in mind and body. Will your memory be the same as it was before menopause? No. You will have a newer type of memory in that the speed with which you think and remember things will not be as fast as it was before. Without the effects of estrogen, you can still have a keen, sharp memory. (See "Normal Aging" below.)

However, some people, if Alzheimer's disease runs in the family, simply can't tolerate the brain fog at menopause. So they may need to try bioidentical estrogen replacement. If this is you, a note of concern. If you are 40 or more pounds overweight, understand that your body already has excessive tissue stores of estrogen. Even if someone has checked your salivary and blood levels of estrogen, the estrogen that can increase your chance toward endometrial and breast cancer isn't stored in the blood and saliva, as we saw in Chapter 1; it's stored in body fat. Look in the mirror. You know where your body fat is. It's in your abdomen. It's in your pelvic area, and it's in your breast area. Women who are 40 pounds or more overweight postmenopausally have an increased risk for breast and endometrial cancer, so if this is you, and you have this brain fog, you may want to consider other ways of dealing with your memory symptoms. You need to know that estrogen replacement alone does not prevent Alzheimer's disease.

You also need to know that for many people, no amount of midlife bioidentical estrogen replacement gets rid of depression or anxiety, so if either of these mood changes is clouding your memory (see the next section in this clinic), you need to aggressively consider treating your brain with nutritional supplements, medicines, and other therapies to elevate your mood and make you calmer.

In addition, you may want to consider looking at other causes of temporary memory loss. The most common causes of confusional state or brain fog are nutritional deficiencies like B12 folate. People who have anemia, hypoglycemia, or problems with emphysema, COPD, or asthma also often have this kind of fuzz-ball brain. Alcohol or drugs often create brain fog, and this often can get confused with memory problems like Alzheimer's disease. If you're taking a variety of antidepressants, antihypertensive meds, beta-blockers, or antihistamines (Benadryl), they too might fog your memory. Check your B6, B12, and folate levels: B6, B12, and folate help your brain make serotonin, a neurotransmitter that's important for mood, anxiety, attention, and memory. If you are using alcohol to treat insomnia, it can make your memory worse; ask your doctor for other nutritional supplements, herbs, and medicines to help you get to sleep. And if you have suffered and continue to suffer from pain or allergies, have a pharmacist or doctor look over your medicines to find out if they too can be causing you to have depression, memory problems, or both.

NORMAL AGING

What's the difference between normal aging and Alzheimer's disease? In Alzheimer's disease, the brain degenerates, and there is a buildup of plaques and tangles in the hippocampus and specific networks throughout the brain. Some forms of Alzheimer's disease that develop early in life are genetic, related to the APOE4 gene. Yes, the same gene that's related to cholesterol and heart disease. Yes, there may be a connection between cholesterol, heart disease, and your risk for Alzheimer's disease. But the majority of Alzheimer's disease is not genetic. If Alzheimer's disease develops later in life, it's related to multiple factors, including environmental toxins, disease, stress, and physical and emotional trauma.

We are capable of aging normally, and the aging brain normally has a potential for lifelong learning. The function of all our brains is to accumulate knowledge over time and to benefit from experience.[5] Yes, it's true, some of us lose brain cells as we get older, but you've been doing that since you were born. Like a potter removing inessential pieces of clay when he or she molds a vase, in a process called apoptosis our brain has been programmed since birth to cut out connections that muddy our thinking. You know what it's like to talk to people who include a lot of inessential details when they talk. They go on this tangent, that tangent. Their mind is cloudy. Your brain is programmed to get rid of these details, nonessential connections, so the wisdom can shine through. So the vast majority of our brain cells we keep and need to protect, cherish, and nourish with food, learning, and healthy relationships. However, the longer we live, the longer we are exposed to environmental toxins, disease, stress, and trauma. So we all need mechanisms to neutralize the effects of the slings and arrows, the ups and downs of living life on planet Earth. Incidentally, as long as you're on Earth, wear a helmet when you ride a bike.

So, it is true that as you get older, you have an increased risk for vulnerability to dementia and the risk increases as you age.[6] However, normal aging involves an increased amount of connections between our brain cells, an increase in wiring between the areas of your brain into your 70s and later. Most people think that part of normal aging is to lose your memory, but that's far from true.[7]

DEMENTIA-PROOF YOUR BRAIN

All of us have a capacity to age into magnificence. There is some variation in how people age. Not everybody has the same set of misfortunes throughout their lives.[8] Some people have more stress, and some people have better skills to handle the stress they have. Some people have better diets; some people have had more environmental toxins. Other people have more resilience to handle and reframe their unique tragedies and traumas. But all of us have a capacity as we age to learn and to change via plasticity in our brain. You can change and turn around what's happened to you all the way to your 70s, 80s, 90s, and later. Who knows? It's not true that an old dog can't learn new tricks. Do they really study old dogs? I don't think so. In fact, they've studied teaching *people* with mild to moderate dementia how to learn: they teach them how to learn new things, and their dementia actually improves.

So how can you dementia-proof your brain?

- First, address lifelong depression and grief. If you've had a lot of loss in your life, get a counselor, someone who can be supportive. Like Susan, you need to have somebody sit with you, listen to you as you talk through and release the grief. If you sit with grief for a long time and it marinates in your body, it eats up neurotransmitters, increases inflammation in your blood vessels, and can set the scene for a variety of degenerative disorders in your body, not to mention dementia. Release the need to immerse yourself in taking care of anybody and everybody to escape your grief. Yeah, you may feel better by being something to everybody. Being alone with one's grief is always hard. Immersing yourself in the thrill and the ecstasy of rescuing can after a while be an addiction and an escape. So get support to release the grief before it becomes a major depression. Long-term depression and its release of cortisol can have an ill effect on your brain's memory circuits.

- If you can't get to sleep, have a doctor or a nurse practitioner help you with nutritional medicines, supplements, herbs or other substances. Now is not the time to sit up at night. You need as much REM as you can get, because REM is how your brain makes acetylcholine, that critical neurotransmitter for sleep.[9] Yes, you remember me saying this earlier in the chapter. I'm saying it twice because it's important.

- Don't take too much vitamin A or D, even though you've heard that it can lower your risk for cancer, because, ironically, excessive amounts of these fat-soluble vitamins may impair your memory. And while you're at it, have someone check your kidney and liver function, as well as your blood sugar, to make sure these are not imbalanced because these are subtle forms of changes in the biochemistry of your brain and body that may make you feel like you have brain fog. Now is the time to get a regular coach to help you get exercise every day. It will help you get blood flow in the blood vessels in your brain and will help encourage healthier blood pressure. Regular exercise will lower your blood sugar, lower your risk for diabetes, and, once again, lower your risk for blood vessel–related dementia, so-called multi-infarct dementia.

- Consider taking an aspirin a day, as it too will inhibit those small artery strokes in your brain that can cause memory loss. Talk to your health care practitioner first to find out if it's safe.

- If you're already taking a statin to lower your cholesterol, consider coenzyme Q10 400 to 600 milligrams a day, as statins are notorious for lowering coenzyme Q10.

Consider also the following laundry list of supplements that can sharpen your mind and sharpen your memory:

- Acetyl-l-carnitine 500 milligrams three times a day—an antioxidant, it protects your brain cells from brain death. It doesn't just sharpen your mind and focus and attention; it can help people who already have mild to moderate Alzheimer's disease have improvement in their memory.

- CDP choline 500 to 2,000 milligrams a day— although controversial, it helps your brain make that neurotransmitter for memory, acetylcholine. CDP choline is considered a cognitive enhancer. It may repair nerve cell membranes that have already been damaged by trauma, stroke, toxins, and aging.

- Vitamin E 2,000 IU.

- DHA 1,000 milligrams three times a day. Fish oil may help people with mild cognitive impairment and milder forms of dementia and may improve short-term and working memory.[10]

- Folic acid 0.8 milligrams a day, B6 20 milligrams a day, B12 0.5 milligrams a day may minimize the shrinkage of the volume of a brain, especially in the memory areas that tend to shrink in Alzheimer's disease.[11]

- L-methyl folate 5.6 mg, methylcobalamin, and N-acetyl-cysteine 600 milligrams—all have been shown to be helpful in those who are concerned about early memory loss or those who tend to have those small strokes in their brain.

- Bioidentical estrogen—talk to your doctor about the risk of breast or endometrial cancer in you or someone in your family. If you have already had breast, ovarian, or endometrial cancer, you may want to avoid hormones entirely, but ultimately the decision is between you and your physician.

- Siberian ginseng—625 milligrams once a day may help your brain release acetylcholine, the memory neurotransmitter, as well as helping protect the nerve cells in your brain.

- Ginkgo biloba—120 to 240 milligrams a day helps with people who are middle-aged with mild memory complaints. It also helps increase acetylcholine levels and improves memory and attention.

- Zinc, selenium, and alpha-tocotrienol help prevent those inflammation changes in the brain by "sucking up" free radicals that may cause nerve cell death in Alzheimer's disease.

AGING WITH POTENTIAL AND PURPOSE

To protect your brain against dementia, it's also important to create growth, change, and lifelong learning. Make sure you're learning in multiple areas in your life. And this is not just about doing the crossword puzzles or Sudoku. Whether it's learning language, honing a three-dimensional sense like learning how to navigate with a map, or doing puzzles, it's important to challenge yourself in multiple realms, whether on planet Earth or otherwise.

Don't get stuck in a rut with just the friends you have. Widen your circle. Join the Y. Get involved in some team sports, even if you've never been much of a "team player." Take a dance class even though up to this point you've kind of had two left feet.

Change how you organize and plan your house. If you're "a creature of habit," change it. You don't want to get cognitive rigidity, do you? Or "hardening of the attitude"? Hire someone to come into your house and change your sock drawer. Change the organization of your closet, even if it means putting all the hangers facing in the opposite direction (and believe me, I don't like this any more than you do!).

Start getting different magazines. If you've always gotten *The Boston Globe*, get *The New York Times*. Yes, the print will be smaller— too bad! Get a magnifying glass. If you've always read hardcover books, get a Kindle. If you're technology-phobic, get your local teenager to teach you. Don't say, "Oh, I don't do technology." You want to follow along with the rest of the herd, because if the rest of the world is doing it, you don't want to be left behind, do you? Learning means exercising the cells in your hippocampus, and that is an anti-dementia behavior. If all the kids in your family or your neighborhood are getting PlayStations or Xboxes or the latest video game, consider learning how to use one, or even buy one. At first you'll feel ridiculous. You may even feel cognitively challenged when you first try to use the controller. It will be particularly annoying when you see an 8-year-old or a 12-year-old use the same machine with no problem whatsoever. However, consider the medicinal effects of laying down new pathways in your brain. The immense effort you will expend, not to mention pushing through embarrassment, will be worth its weight in gold as you lower your risk for dementia. You would be pleased to know that I'm on my third PlayStation and I also carry a Game Boy. People look at me strangely. I don't care. Learn a different language. Learn Spanish. Try to learn a different alphabet. Yes, it is painfully difficult. Do it anyway. Listen and talk to someone with a different political bent. This may be painfully difficult too. Notice I didn't say necessarily change your political attitudes; I said, listen and consider what other people are saying. Try to wrap your mind around how they came to that point of view.

Volunteering at a nearby shelter area where a lot of minorities tend to cluster can help you learn different languages that are spoken. You'll learn one sentence or one phrase here or there, and you'll become in essence a polyglot. If you are losing your hearing, get fitted with a hearing aid. If you're losing your eyesight, figure out a different way of seeing, even if it means Braille. If you're losing a sense, your chance of dementia skyrockets. If you can't hear, now is not the time to say you don't want to look old because you have a hearing aid.

Rent a car and drive yourself around, because it will help you practice three-dimensional skills. So you get lost! You may find yourself in an amazing place. Pull over; get a great meal in a place you would never have gone. Don't be afraid to make mistakes and meet new people. Mingle with local spiritual groups, recreational groups, occupational groups.

Don't retire. This is a big one. People will say, "But I've worked long and hard. I deserve to retire." The literature suggests that retirement increases your risk within five years of developing dementia, cancer, heart disease, and stroke. Instead of saying you're retiring, say, "I'm ending this career and choosing another avocation or calling." I'm not saying substitute another nine-to-five job; however, puttering around the house or waiting for your partner to be available to do something with you is a pro-dementia track.

Hang out with people who are a variety of ages. Yes, you may be uncomfortable at first—you know the saying "Birds of a feather flock together." You don't want to be birds of a feather dementing together, though. By being with children along with adults, you'll be made to move faster and keep up. And for the people who are older, you'll want to help them speed up. Multigenerational activities are the best to help you maintain flexibility in your brain and your body.[12]

II. Anxiety, Trauma, and Memory

Did you have emotional or physical trauma in your childhood? Are you having problems now in your family relationships, finances, and work? If so, the stress hormones of cortisol and epinephrine may increase your chance toward having problems with your memory. If you'll *remember*, there are two types of memory. There is the hippocampus, the area that lays down memory we can talk about, and then there's the other type of memory. The amygdala is body memory. The amygdala takes over for the hippocampus when events around you are overwhelmingly panicking, terrorizing, distressing, and catastrophic. During trauma, the amygdala funnels panic and anger to your body via the hypothalamus and hormones. The result? When you're in a traumatic situation now, first you feel panic and anger, then numbness. However, over time, if the trauma is unrelenting, hypothalamus and hormones transform the pain into body memories. And then, later on in your life, if you are in a situation that is reminiscent of the past trauma, you may be blissfully and blithely unaware. However, your body won't be.

Medical-intuitively, even if you think that partner or neighborhood or family feels like "home," it may actually match that oh-so-familiar traumatic memory of what home was like. You may feel an. initial emotional comfort and familiarity, but your body won't. Medical-intuitively, your body will sound an alarm of warning to multiple organs, letting you know to reconsider the safety of your situation. It is possible that those of us who've experienced trauma may have a lifelong distorted vision, a blindness toward knowing what a safe family is if we've had an abusive one. We may not be able to accurately see a safe relationship if we've had a series of abusive ones. And we may have a similar myopic visual incapacity to see what could be vocationally possible if we've had a series of jobs in which we've had abusive bosses or even been fired.

So what do you do if the memory circuits in your brain and body have been altered by trauma? In addition to the solutions in the following section, you may, like anyone who has physical blindness, borrow a pair of eyes for that area of your life. You may for the rest of your life need to borrow someone's perceptivity and wisdom in seeing what *is* a healthy group of people to be in. You may need the balanced perspective of a coach or psychotherapist, like a Seeing Eye dog, to help guide you and support you to choose appropriate mates and careers. Is it possible, through psychotherapy and "working through our issues," that we can say to ourselves, "By now, after decades of making the same relationship or career mistakes, I should be able to choose more wisely"? Perhaps. There are two ways of looking at this. Until you get there, you may still need the visual support of a counselor to help guide you to make the correct choices, because if you continue to make the wrong, trauma-inducing choices, you drive memory problems further into your brain and body. However, in people who have the most severe traumatic pasts, science shows us that there may be a more extensive rearrangement of vision and memory circuits in their brains for recognizing relationships and opportunities accurately. So part of aging wisely is to accept one's limits gracefully as one learns to acquire new talents. For example, Stevie Wonder is blind and in his 70s at the time of this writing. Perhaps his blindness, in his brain, may have made him lose visual capabilities but develop lifelong savant gifts for melody and musical genius. The man is blind. You wouldn't think he would say, "Any day now, through the right amount of psychotherapy, I'm going to see, because I've 'worked through' the problem."

That opens up another whole can of worms. We can deal with trauma's effects in our brain and body, and perhaps even eradicate, cure, heal, and remove certain illnesses. However, we can never really remove our memory of its effects on our life, traumatic or otherwise. Having experienced all of those events, painful or otherwise, affects our brain and may in fact impact our memory in just the way we're talking about in this story. So accepting what has happened to you and loving yourself for the person you've created to endure the trauma, the only way you're going to help your memory is to *accept* help.

Consider the following questions to find out if you've experienced anxiety and trauma that affects your memory circuits.

EMOTIONAL SYMPTOMS

- There have been long periods of time in your life when you've experienced nervousness and worry to such a level that you can hardly stand it.

- There's been an event or events in your life in which you've experienced such terror that you wondered how you would survive.

- There's been an event or events in your life in which you've watched the tragedy of a close loved one experiencing a horrific trauma and felt powerless and guilty because you couldn't help them.

BODY SYMPTOMS

- Since you can remember, your body has had hot flashes and cold chills.

- Since you can remember, you've had episodes in which your chest tends to pound.

- You've had long periods of time in your life where you've had problems with dizziness and lightheadedness.

- For long periods of time, you've wondered if your nervous system was keyed up; your body felt trembling, shaking, sometimes numbness and tingling.

- For most of your life it's been hard for you to swallow pills.

- You get a lot of side effects from medicines, herbs, and nutritional supplements.

Only you can determine how many of the above symptoms of nervousness and anxiety may be making it harder for you to remember. If you are a high-strung person who has emotional and intuitive hypersensitivity, your edginess and tension may make your memory perform less efficiently than it can. Anxiety, however, may be only one component of what is making you struggle to have efficient, sharp memory. After you read the following case, read the other sections in this chapter as well, as they may help you find other solutions to utilize all of your intellect and wisdom.

TERRY: TRAUMA AND MEMORY

Terry, 58, called me complaining that she couldn't remember anything. She said her brain was in a fog.

THE INTUITIVE READING

When I looked at Terry's life, I saw that after she lost a loved one in her life, she seemed to always be nervous about being alone. Was it a parent? Did someone just up and leave the family? Whatever it was, it seemed that Terry's brain and body had a hypervigilance, a twitchy sense that the world was not safe and at any time someone could just go poof and leave her. And now recently, it seemed like her life was on instant replay of this trauma. Someone had again left Terry. This in itself wasn't a tragedy, but it seemed to be compounded because it reminded her of that earlier separation in her life. It felt like Terry had experienced "emotional whiplash."

THE BODY

When I looked at Terry's head, I saw problems with focus and attention. Were these due to hormones? Were they due to panic? I saw pressure in her chest. It was hard to take a deep breath. It seemed that addiction ran in the people around Terry. Was it alcohol? Food? I wasn't sure. I saw subtle changes in estrogen, progesterone, and cortisol and insulin that made her brain fog worse. Finally, I saw sadness and problems falling asleep and staying asleep.

THE FACTS

Terry worked as an interior designer, and it was taking her longer and longer to complete her projects. People were beginning to complain. She couldn't keep to her schedule and was starting to forget some of the details of her assignments. Her mother had died of breast cancer when she was four, and recently her father had died suddenly of a massive heart attack. Terry told me she could remember very little of her childhood, so she really didn't think the death of her mother was that much of a problem. She did admit that she had been in recovery for alcohol for 20 years, having used it for anxiety and insomnia. Recently, she was in perimenopause and was having trouble sleeping. Having long had problems with relationships, she always thought the only thing she could really trust was her success in work, but recently that too was failing her.

THE SOLUTION

If you have had serious trauma in your life, you may have been diagnosed with PTSD, anxiety, depression, and maybe even ADHD. If that's the case, get a neuropsychological assessment for memory, so they can tease out which aspects of your memory issues are due to anxiety, and which ones are due to frontal executive function problems, ADHD, and/or PTSD. The neuropsychologist will be able to give you cognitive remediation for all these disorders. For more solutions, see Chapter 1 on depression, Chapter 2 on anxiety and PTSD, and Chapter 4 on ADHD.

The first solution to trauma to the brain and its effect on memory is certainly not to keep digging it up. Like picking a scab, the more you pick at it, the deeper the scar goes. In addition, trying to remember the traumatic event doesn't necessarily help you heal. It doesn't. Although knowing what happened to you, and how it's influenced your brain, mood, and relationships, may be comforting and informative, it doesn't give you the skills to avoid making the same choice over and over again. The more you unearth a trauma over a series of years by talking about it or repeating it, like a moth attracted to a flame, you'll become hardwired in your brain to repeat it. The more you talk about the trauma over the course of decades, the stronger the memory traces in your brain and body get, increasing the chance that you will unwittingly and unconsciously find yourself unable to make healthier choices in relationships, finances, and work. You're going to need specialized mind-body cognitive behavioral or dialectical behavioral therapy to break the cycle between trauma, the amygdala, habits, and health. Otherwise, your life script will be a bad soap opera, and your health will let you know that you are falling into that dangerous rut again through the symptom of that chronic illness.

EMDR can also be helpful for people who have had trauma. Somehow it may alter how the brain processes memory of painful events. You can use supplements, traditional herbs, and medicines to treat the anxiety, such as ashwagandha, rhodiola, 5-HTP, or others (see Chapter 2). In addition, you might want to consider passion flower or lemon balm to help you get to sleep, not to mention magnesium. Aggressively treat depression (see Chapter 1) with supplements or medicines, as chronic depression can further unhinge the frontal lobe executive function of your brain and make it hard for you to retrieve memory. (See the previous case.)

THE AFFIRMATIONS

Louise Hay has written book after book about how a person forgives after being hurt by a mother, a father, a boss, a friend, a sister, a lover, and so on. She says, "I know you want everybody and everything else to change. It doesn't work that way. If you've been hurt in the past, and you want to change your life, then you are the one that must do the changing." So, according to Louise, if you want to heal trauma, you can't look back to your family, your friends, or the people who have abused you. And, yes, it would be wonderful if they were to apologize, but often a simple apology, or a protracted apology, doesn't make it better, now does it? It really doesn't. The person who has to do the changing to heal is actually you, the one who was hurt. To heal from a trauma, to clear up your mind so that the pain from the injury isn't reverberating over and over and over again, you have to create the changes in your belief, according to Louise. It's not always easy, however. She says, "Life is very simple. What we give out, we get back." Our subconscious mind accepts whatever we choose to believe. Remember, we are dealing with thoughts, and thoughts can be changed. When we were children, we learned about ourselves, about our lives, from the reactions of the adults around us. So, think about it. If you were abused, if you were injured, you're gonna think, *I'm worthy of being abused. I'm not lovable.* You can change that now in the present. That was then and this is now.

Louise goes on, "When we grow up, we have a tendency to re-create the emotional environment of our early home life. We tend to re-create in our personal relationships those we had with our mother and father. If we were highly criticized as children, then we will seek out those in our adult life who will duplicate this behavior. If we were praised, loved, and encouraged as children, then we re-create this behavior. Do not blame your parents." She encourages, "We are all victims of victims and, somehow, they probably were victimized too. They could not teach you something they did not know. If your mother or father did not know how to love themselves, it would have been impossible for them to teach you how to love yourself. They were coping as best as they could with the information they had." Think about it for a minute, how they were raised. If you want to understand your parents more, I suggest you ask them about their childhoods. Listen to not only what they are telling you, but notice what happens while they are speaking. What is their body language like? As you're doing this, I might add, it does not take away from your own anger. It does not invalidate the pain of your trauma. You can do the exercise of seeing your victimizer's experience and at the same time be present for your own pain, anger, and suffering. That's what the *di* is in dialectical behavioral therapy. Di means two—being able to see two apparently paradoxical perspectives at one time.

The innermost belief for everyone is "I am not good enough," and we all suffer from self-hatred and guilt to one degree or another. These are the problems that all of us struggle with in our lives. If we spend our time blaming others and not taking responsibility for our own experiences in the present, we're going to have trouble healing. You can't change your path, but you can change your attitude about the past. What happened to you, happened to you. Past tense. It cannot be changed. But you can change your thoughts about the past, and your reaction to the past, and how it affects how you feel about yourself. And the only road to healing, whether it's brain fog or pain in your body, is through forgiveness. You set the other people free and you set yourself free.

Louise suggests doing the deservability exercise from her mirror work, saying in the mirror, "I am deserving. I deserve all good. Not some, not a little, but *all* good. I now move past all negative and restricting thoughts. I release and let go of the limitations of my parents. I love them. I go beyond them. I am not their negative opinions or limiting beliefs. I am not bound by any of their fears or prejudice. In my mind I have total freedom. I now move in a new space of consciousness. The universe is more than willing to manifest my new belief. I accept this abundant life with joy, pleasure, and gratitude, for I am deserving. I accept it. I know it to be free."

III. ACCIDENTS, CONCUSSION, BRAIN INJURY, AND MEMORY

We've been falling on our heads since childhood when we took our first steps. It's a normal function of our brain and body to repair after injury, whether it's a scrape on our knee, a broken bone here and there, or even a mild bang to your head when you fall off the swing set or go over the handlebars of your bike. Your body and brain can be incredibly forgiving after insult or injury, emotional or physical trauma.

What makes an injury, a blow to our head, give us problems with memory? A variety of factors, including our genetics, our nutritional status, and whether or not we use alcohol or drugs. However, we cannot minimize the influence that our environment or our behavior has on our capacity to come back, rewire our brains, and compensate after an injury: whether we grew up with an intense desire to learn or were not in an environment where learning was encouraged, whether we have resources such as nutritional supplements, herbs, medicines, and a variety of therapies. The impact that an injury has on the brain isn't the same from one person to another.

What is brain injury anyway? In its mildest form, a concussion is a traumatic brain injury in which a sudden force is directed against one's head, face, or neck. Whether it occurs in a car accident, an athletic event, or another injury, there are classical symptoms and signs: a loss of consciousness, irritability, slow reaction times, drowsiness, headache, brain fog, emotional lability, are but a few of the symptoms. The symptoms of concussions usually resolve on their own; however, many concussions aren't even recognized as having occurred by the person who is injured.

In the United States alone, 1.7 million people have a traumatic brain injury of one kind or another each year. Most people don't seek medical advice, but for those who do, the total cost of their care in the U.S. alone in the year 2000 was $60 billion.[13]

If you're concerned that an injury to your head, be it from a slip or a fall, an athletic injury or a car accident, has affected your memory, go the emergency room immediately after it happens. The doctors and nurses on staff will provide the proper exams and scans and other tests to determine the severity of your injury, not to mention the proper treatment and follow-up. If months later you find you're "still not right," having brain fog, memory problems, or other symptoms, consider going to a neurologist and getting a neuropsychological assessment for attention, learning, and memory. Those professionals will be able to take a "neuropsychiatric snapshot" of how your brain is functioning now to see what the basis is for your memory complaints.

Other than the symptoms of concussion that we just described, what are some of the other brain problems one may have after one or more injuries? Many of the symptoms come under the heading of the frontal lobe brain area, that area we described in Chapter 4 on learning disorders.

- As you might recall, the frontal lobe's executive area functions to curb, censor, direct, and organize your temporal lobe limbic areas for emotion. So someone who's had perhaps a more extensive brain injury may experience some personality changes, since the frontal lobe and the temporal lobe work together to shape our personality and how we act and behave.

- Sometimes after a more extensive brain injury, injury to the frontal lobe removes the usual inhibition that we need to curb impulses, whether it's at work, in relationships, in finances, or in families. Someone who's had a brain injury may impulsively respond to a stray comment with irritability, moodiness, and then depression.

- Someone who was previously anxious or sensitive may, after a brain injury, have exaggerated panic after a seemingly mild scare or in an unfamiliar situation. Someone with a brain injury simply can't stop talking about that terror. They will not just ruminate about it like someone who's obsessional or compulsive (see

Chapter 2); they will "perseverate," that is, be unable to get off the topic and keep coming back to it over and over again, no matter how much family members, mates, or colleagues try to change the subject.

- After brain injury, the frontal lobe "brake" may make it hard for someone to control their temper or their mood. Someone who was previously a more or less even-keeled individual may, after a brain injury, find themselves flying off the handle more easily. Impatient, irritable, you may find yourself flying off the handle if someone cuts you off in traffic, takes too long in front of you in the checkout line, or even makes too much noise.

- After a traumatic brain injury, the frontal lobe's attention and organization areas may not work as efficiently. Even if you previously had a lot of motivation and initiative, after a series of concussions or injuries you may find it hard to be as productive as you used to be, engage with friends and family, in travel or entertainment; your body may feel like lead. You may get lost in a morass of details at work and find it hard to organize your job, your shopping, or even plans for a trip.

- And finally, when it comes to your memory, you may notice (or others may notice even more than you do) that you're not as "sharp" as you used to be. During a conversation, when someone is talking to you, you may remember only a detail here or there from what they've said, while friends and family who are listening at the same time seem to be getting so much more out of the conversation. Unless you take notes or write down what you've heard, if anything is told to you, it goes in one ear and out the other. You simply can't remember it.

If you have any or all of these symptoms, after you've gone for a neuropsychological evaluation, read on to the following case study. Don't get discouraged. Brain injury is oh so common. So many famous people who function quite successfully have had bad accidents with this injury, and they have learned all the ways to nourish and supplement their brain to function well. You can too. You can heal your mind, even after brain injury, to create wholeness with medicine, affirmations, and intuition.

VIVIAN: A BLOW TO THE HEAD

Vivian, age 38, called me with concerns about hormones.

THE INTUITIVE READING

When I looked at Vivian, she seemed like the epitome of health. She never seemed to complain of health problems. Vivian seemed strong, with an indomitable spirit. I wondered why she was even calling me for a reading.

THE BODY

When I looked at her head, I immediately understood why. It was like a dense fog. I saw problems with focus, attention, and distractibility. I saw Vivian having problems at work with her judgment. I could just see her spend too much time on a detail that was inconsequential while blowing off the most important part of the project. In addition to having problems with priorities and judgment, Vivian also seemed distracted, so much so that she was having problems finishing projects entirely. Was it because she was having difficulty working in a crowded environment where there was noise and distraction? And although I saw that she was extremely creative, with a strong intellect, I wondered if it was hard for her to access it through this dense fog in her head. Beyond the fog, there were a few musculoskeletal issues in her neck and ribs. Were these athletic injuries? Accidents?

THE FACTS

Vivian told me that she was very healthy and a runner, and, yes, she'd had an injury here or there. She was concerned about getting her hormones stable, but no matter what doctors did, they couldn't balance her estrogen and progesterone. When Vivian didn't immediately talk about brain fog, I instead asked her about whether she'd had any accidents or injuries. She said, "Oh, that's that car accident I had when I was 17, and I was in a coma for two weeks." A coma for *two weeks*? "Yes," she said. "I had a fracture in my skull, and the doctors put in a metal plate." She said after that, she was fine. I asked her how far she had gone in school; she told me that after the accident she'd tried to go back and finish college, but she couldn't. Since that time, she'd had a series of jobs, many of which she'd either been laid off from or left before she could be fired due to some "misunderstanding." Vivian said that working in an office was never her thing anyway. She had a tendency to be porous and sensitive and easily distracted in a busy office environment. Now she worked for an elderly lawyer, and she was able to do her work at home. But lately, at perimenopause, even with these work adaptations, she was finding herself with her hormonal issues still not being able to focus.

TRAUMATIC BRAIN INJURY AND MEMORY

Whether brain injury is mild, moderate, or severe, two injuries occur in the brain in varying amounts. First, when force is applied to your head, the brain hits the skull and it wiggles around. As the brain wiggles, connections between the brain cells—axons—are stretched to varying degrees and then become disconnected from each other. This process is called diffuse axonal injury, and it may be the cause of much of what people experience after a concussion. The headaches, the fatigue, the problems with concentration, slow thinking, forgetfulness, dizziness, light-headedness, depression with insomnia, irritability.

On the other hand, in more severe forms of brain injury, more dramatic changes in the structure of the brain take place. Along the pathways in the brain, there are arteries. In more severe brain injury, when those nerve cell pathways get stretched and injured, the arteries also become injured, and they can bleed. This bleeding can cause inflammation over time, and in some people (not all) the inflammation can cause degeneration and memory loss.

For a long time, doctors didn't understand the level of brain anatomy changes that occur in the mildest forms of brain injury.[14] However, now, newer technology, such as diffusion tensor imagery (DTI) and tractography, shows that people with these syndromes actually have abnormalities in these white matter connection pathways. These very subtle changes that occur in mild brain injury may be underlying the symptoms that occur, including depression, irritability, anxiety, and brain fog.[15]

If you have had multiple concussions over time, you need to be specially careful about engaging in athletic events or taking risks that may subject your brain to further injury. In some individuals, if you have multiple concussions over time, you can develop a disorder called chronic traumatic encephalopathy (CTE). In chronic traumatic encephalopathy, one's problem is not merely the blow to the head. After multiple hits to the brain, multiple small concussions, a chronic inflammation occurs along brain pathways. Inflammatory mediators are released. Inflammation can occur months, years, or even decades after the brain trauma. These brain changes may affect memory and judgment, cause confusion and problems controlling impulse, aggression, and even cause dementia. Originally, we thought CTE was the progressive degenerative disorder that only boxers had. We called it dementia pugilistica, because boxers had multiple concussions from being hit in the head. However, now we know that any number of individuals can have CTE, in the National Football League, ice hockey, wrestling, soccer, and so on. Domestic violence is also being investigated in this regard. Interestingly, when you examine the brains of people who have had multiple concussions over time, you may see nerve cell loss or tau protein, as well as beta-amyloid and neurofibrillary tangles. These are among the same markers we see in individuals with other dementing disorders, such as Alzheimer's disease.

As I said earlier, when you've had a brain injury, the first step is to get an immediate evaluation and treatment. Go immediately to the hospital emergency room and get the appropriate scan. You want to make sure you don't have the bleeding vessels that are associated with head injuries. But on the other hand, if you do have a head injury, you want to immediately start to heal your mind with everything available, whether it's nutritional supplements, herbs, medicines, or a variety of healing remedies. You want to consider everything that's available to feel whole again.

THE SUPPLEMENTS

After you've dealt with the emergency situation, it's important that you use nutritional supplements and herbs to help nourish your brain away from the inflammation. Though many of these solutions may be controversial and not fully studied yet, I wouldn't wait until the studies come in. I would talk to my treatment team about taking coenzyme Q10, an anti-inflammatory, 400 to 600 milligrams a day. I would use supplements and medicines, especially antioxidants such as:

- Alpha-tocotrienol, a high potency anti-inflammatory
- A baby aspirin a day, but only if your doctor says it's okay
- Acetyl-L-carnitine 500 milligrams two or three times a day, which is a neuroprotective and also has an antioxidant effect and prevents cell death
- CDP choline 500 to 2,000 milligrams a day, which helps you maintain the building blocks for acetyl choline, that critical memory neurotransmitter
- Tomato, potato, or eggplant—eating these can theoretically increase acetylcholine in your brain
- Siberian ginseng if your blood pressure is normal (625 milligrams once a day)

- If you're not worried about bleeding, and if your doctor says it's okay, ginkgo biloba 120 to 240 milligrams a day

- To maintain acetylcholine, huperzine A 60 to 200 micrograms per day

- SAMe, but only if you're not using other serotonin medicines; 400 milligrams two to three times a day on an empty stomach, otherwise it doesn't work

- A multivitamin that has B6, B12, and folic acid, all of which help your brain make serotonin; they also decrease levels of the inflammatory mediator homocysteine

- DHA 1,000 milligrams three times a day

- Phosphatidylserine, although controversial, 100 to 300 milligrams a day

OTHER APPROACHES

If you have had brain injury of any kind, I think it's important to reevaluate the state of your brain function. Consider getting a neuropsychological assessment for frontal executive function, attention, learning, and memory, especially if your concussion symptoms haven't improved after six months. If your memory symptoms have affected your capacity for work and relationships, have the neuropsychologist refer you to appropriate cognitive behavioral therapy, vocational therapy, and other support to help you adapt while you recover from your injury.[16]

Also, I would learn, learn, learn, learn, learn. I would put myself in an information-rich environment. I would try to read the newspaper in print or online every day. (I emphasize *try*.) You may not feel you are remembering all of it, but right now that's not what's important. What's important is that you are subjecting your brain to literary information and exercising your language circuits. Even if you read one paragraph or two paragraphs a day, or just read the headlines, you are pumping neurons in your brain and exercising your attention and memory circuits.

But most important, I would remove myself from an environment where my head was going to get hit. If you are a football player, stop. If you are a soccer player, stop. Right now, we don't have helmets that are going to save your head. If you continue to play the same sport professionally, you are essentially mortgaging your brain for the sake of your bank account.

Try meditation and yoga to lower cortisol, the stress neurotransmitter. Use acupuncture to increase cerebral blood flow to areas in your brain.

Although controversial, hyperbaric oxygen a decade ago was being used by people with traumatic brain injury. This therapy is now used "off label" for a variety of scenarios, including Asperger's, autism, and others. New studies suggest that when compared with a placebo, hyperbaric oxygen has little effect. New research is being done, however, showing that soldiers with blast injuries in war may be helped with hyperbaric oxygen.[17]

If you've had a moderate to severe brain injury, you want to check your hormone levels: TSH, T4, T3 and other hormones, and especially testosterone, estrogen, and progesterone. A more severe blow to your head could affect the connections between your brain, hypothalamus, and pituitary, making your hormones erratic. And while we're on the subject of hormones, although progesterone has not been considered to be helpful, beta estradiol and amantadine immediately after an injury have been shown to significantly decrease cell death. So if you haven't had cancer, or if cancer doesn't run in your family, you might want to consider talking to a complementary doctor about whether you are a candidate for these kinds of treatment.[18]

What about biofeedback? Believe it or not, biofeedback, that is, working with heart rate variability, has been helpful for people with brain injury, even severe brain injury. These kinds of treatments not only improve social functioning but have also been shown to improve emotional symptoms.[19]

And then there's laser therapy. Some newer research suggests that people with mild brain injury have been helped with lasers, specifically transcranial near-infrared light. Not only does this therapy improve cognitive performance, it helps with frontal lobe function, distractibility, and problems with organization and planning.[20]

Is the future now? There are new treatment approaches to brain injury that are being researched now. Scientists are working aggressively on stem cell transplants for brain injury.[21] Then there are the drugs. Some newer drugs that work at the glutamate receptor may be particularly helpful for brain injury, as glutamate may be involved with the inflammation cascade that occurs within 24 hours after injury.[22] If I had a relative with a traumatic brain injury, I'd have them consider all of these treatments. I'd suggest acupuncture, Chinese medicine, to stop the inflammatory cascade, as well as ginkgo biloba, curcumin, centella asiatica, any of these anti-inflammatory herbs, not to mention the supplements that may stop chronic inflammation that can occur years down the road.[23] I would suggest hyperbaric oxygen. I would have them exercise their brain and body to learn as much as possible so they could use all of their mind for the rest of their life.

There's nothing new under the sun. Concussions and brain injury aren't new. Perhaps our awareness of them is. On some level we can't prevent an accident. We can brace ourselves with seat belts, but in the end, it's an accident. However, we can buffer our body from the slings and arrows of life, whether with nutritional supplements, herbs, or medicines, believing that against adversity we can be safe and strong.

THE AFFIRMATIONS

Whether it's an accident or an injury, we may all feel anger believing that the accident or the collision, the lack of safe equipment, "shouldn't have happened." Things "should be different." This is "unfair." After the accident, if you've had injuries other than to your brain and memory—maybe injuries to your spine, legs, and so on—you may be bitter at having nearly lost your life, not to mention losing a certain part of your identity, whether it's involved in playing a certain sport or having your body and brain be a certain way. In addition to the physical aftereffects of a brain injury, we have to deal with the depression and bitterness over the fact that life itself has dealt us "a bad hand."

Louise Hay has a forgiveness checklist that may help you move through the anger and trauma after you've had an accident or incident in which somebody else also was involved in the injury to your body and brain. Statements like "I'll never forgive them," "What they did was unforgivable," "They ruined my life," "I don't have to forgive anyone, it's their fault," "They did this to me"— though the statement may be true, you may have been hit by that car or by that bullet or by that fist, feeling self-righteous or carrying a grudge year after year isn't therapeutic. Being angry after your injury and carrying that anger for years on end releases inflammatory mediators in your brain and body, and we already know that brain injury in itself involves inflammatory mediators. You don't need to add more on top of that by maintaining in your mind those thoughts: *I'm right. They're wrong. Things should be different.* Though that stance may be logical, attaching yourself to that emotion of resentment will only injure your brain and body further, not to mention your memory. Instead, consider working with someone who knows dialectical behavioral therapy. Specifically ask them to help you learn the skill of Radical Acceptance, which helps us accept reality the way it is and learn how to handle suffering mindfully. If you are angry after being injured in an accident, a sporting event, or even an abusive situation, get help from a trained professional who is familiar with emotional and physical trauma. If you've had physical abuse in a relationship, the counselor will help you find out what you need to do to become safe. If you've had more severe brain injury, brain injury rehab units often have counselors that help you deal with the emotional fallout, anger, and frustration from your injury.

In addition, Louise Hay suggests using mirror work, especially when we've had trauma where someone has injured us. Look into your eyes in the mirror and say with feeling, "I am willing to forgive." Repeat this several times. What are you feeling? Do you feel stubborn and stuck? Or do you feel open and willing? Just notice your feelings, don't judge them. Breathe deeply a few times and repeat the exercise. Does it feel any different? Then use the following statements.

- If you believe "I'll never forgive them," your affirmation is "This is a new moment. I am free to let go."

- If you believe "They don't deserve to be forgiven," your affirmation is "I forgive whether they deserve it or not."

- If you believe "What they did to me was unforgivable," your affirmation is "I am willing to go beyond my limitations."

- If you believe "They did it on purpose," your affirmation is "They were doing the best they could with the knowledge, understanding, and awareness they had at the time."

- If you believe "They ruined my life," your affirmation is "I take responsibility for my own life. I am free."

- If you believe "I don't have to forgive anyone," your affirmation is "I refuse to limit myself. I am always willing to take the next step."

Whether it's a small blow or a big blow to your brain or your psyche, say to yourself in the mirror, "I give myself permission to let go."

IV. MEMORY DISORDERS, ALZHEIMER'S DISEASE, AND OTHER DEMENTIAS: THERE IS HOPE

Have you noticed a progressive lessening of your ability to remember things? Have you become less alert, less able to handle the anxiety, stress, and sadness in your daily life? In some cases, a progressive decline in your memory that has a great effect on your daily life can be Alzheimer's disease. But there are many other reversible causes of memory loss that can cause the same symptoms. Please make sure you read the first three sections in this chapter before you come to the conclusion that your memory problems may be Alzheimer's disease.

Alzheimer's disease is a gradual loss of several abilities in your brain, not just memory. Whether it's problems with attention, language, or your ability to orient yourself, use judgment, have insight, and make decisions, memory is the symptom most people think about when they worry about Alzheimer's disease. However, there are other forms of dementia. Lewy body dementia, progressive supranuclear palsy, Parkinson's disease, not to mention other neurodegenerative disorders, can all cause one to have a loss of brain function over time.

Many people who find their attention and memory slipping may not have dementia at all. Their memory problems may be due to any of a host of reversible disorders—physical and chemical disorders in their brains and bodies, including:

- Lyme, Herpes zoster, HIV, cancers, lupus, and other infectious diseases can all cause a brain fog. When your immune system is activated, it creates inflammation molecules like IL1, IL6, TNF alpha, and others that "gum up" the memory apparatus. In this case, your problem with memory can be reversible, and if your illness is treated, you can regain your attention, focus, and memory.

- Nutrition, metabolic, and other toxic disorders. Alcohol and pain meds often can cloud one's brain. B12 deficiency, liver disorders, thyroid problems, adrenal gland/cortisol problems, and exposure to heavy metals can "shuffle" the brain's chemistry, cloud consciousness, and make it hard for you to access memory.

- Heart disease and blood vessel problems. If a person has had a stroke, hypertension, and even recent surgery for correcting clogged arteries, we can have a loss of memory.

- Parasites and infections in the brain can also create an immune disorder that disrupts memory. If you are having a problem with brain fog and fatigue, it's really important to have a full medical workup to rule out the reversible causes of memory loss.

Let's say you are particularly concerned about Alzheimer's disease or other dementias because a parent or other close relative developed that disorder. If so, the first thing you'll want to do is go to a neurologist and have them evaluate you for any and all causes of memory problems. Neurologists have a variety of diagnostic instruments fine-tuned to pick up whether or not your memory symptoms may be caused by a neurodegenerative disorder like Alzheimer's disease or other forms of dementia.

However, caution: if you are particularly intellectually gifted and/or have had a lot of education, your memory symptoms may not be picked up by their tests. Why? With years of intellectual enrichment, you may have built in brain circuits that compensate for and cover up your memory symptoms, so standard tests are not going to pick up those subtle symptoms of memory loss that you know are really occurring. If this is you, you will notice that perhaps it's taking oh so much longer to do the *New York Times* crossword puzzle in ink. Or when it comes to preparing four people's tax returns in a weekend, you find that you're not as sharp as you used to be. Normal testing will think you're "being too hard on yourself" and making excessive demands. With such a "high ceiling effect" in how you've trained your brain to perform, it might be better that you go to a neuropsychologist and have them give you a full-scale neuropsychological evaluation. Commensurate with your education and career, a skilled board-certified neuropsychologist will be able to more or less interpret to what degree your memory may have slipped. In the meantime, with help from a friend or loved one, consider the following statements:

- In addition to having problems with your memory, you have a *consistent* problem with your memory and your thinking.

- You have problems remembering recent events, like what you had for dinner the night before or what you did last weekend.

- You have trouble remembering a short shopping list.

- Your memory has especially gone downhill in the last year.

- A partner or family member is also concerned about your memory.

- You have recently forgotten a major event, like a party, wedding, or trip, within a few weeks of the event.

- You have trouble remembering important information about your past, such as your wedding date, your place of employment, and so on.

- Your memory problems are making it hard for you to do your work.

- Your memory problems may have cost you your job or forced you to retire.

If many of these statements seem to fit your experience, then in addition to using the solutions in this book, it's very important that you create a team not just to help you find the source of your memory problems, but to support you day to day. In addition to nutritional supplements, herbs, medicines, and a host of other therapies, you may for the time being need a variety of people to help make sure you're effectively and safely keeping track of the details of your life, whether it's handling finances, responding to household emergencies, or even managing your long-term schedule with your family and friends or at work. Support is something you need right now to effectively navigate the challenges in your brain and body.[24]

Read on to the following story to find out how to manage memory, aging, and concerns about Alzheimer's disease and other dementias.

WHITNEY: NOT JUST TIRED

Whitney said that people were concerned about her memory. She wasn't sure if she had any problems. She just thought she was tired. Whitney's adult daughter sat in on the reading.

THE INTUITIVE READING

When I looked at Whitney's life, it felt like one of those model houses that they have in a new housing development. Everything is staged. Everything is sterile. None of the furniture seems personal. I had a hard time seeing anything personal on the walls of her house as I intuitively looked around. If people's personal effects had been in the house, it was as if they were taken away. I couldn't see a picture of a spouse. I couldn't see pictures of children. Was Whitney experiencing some loss? I could only see the bare-bones evidence of somebody living in a house.

THE BODY

Whitney seemed generally healthy. However, she seemed to be having problems with focus and attention, and there weren't a lot of ideas flowing in her mind. I had a hard time following her train of thought. Usually when I do a reading, I can feel what someone's worried about, whether they're concerned about work, kids, family. However, when it came to Whitney, I couldn't see details about her life flowing in and out of her head. There was just this space, just as uncrowded as the house I saw earlier in the reading.

THE FACTS

Whitney said she had always prided herself on keeping her health and her appearance pristine and staying active. However, lately she had had a series of losses. Her partner had died five years earlier of cancer, and her two children had moved to the other side of the country. She had taken an early retirement package from her teaching job and moved into a retirement community. Since that time, Whitney had felt tired, not really wanting to do activities with the other residents. Soon her family became concerned.

They said there was something different about her conversation. She couldn't get her words out; it seemed like the word she wanted was always on the tip of her tongue.

Whitney did admit that she was hanging out less with people at parties because she was having trouble following conversations. Her family had her check her hearing, but it was normal. Lately she had gotten depressed, overwhelmed, and anxious in the late afternoons. Her family pointed this out to her, but she just thought she was getting tired. Recently, a neurologist told her that her memory showed the very early signs of Alzheimer's disease and suggested medication. Whitney had never taken any medication before, not even for cholesterol or blood pressure, since her health had always been, as I said, pristine. She and her family wanted to know what was available to help "sharpen up" her mind and buffer her brain against possible memory disorders like Alzheimer's disease.

What to Do If You Think You're Losing Your Memory

Go to a neurologist who will evaluate you to find out what is the source of your memory disorder. Whether it's injury (as in the last case), nutritional problems, or body chemical abnormalities, the physician will tease out the multiple factors that are unraveling your memory networks. In addition, the memory team may be able to determine if depression (as in section I of this clinic), anxiety (section II), or trauma (section III) further contributes to your memory loss. They will evaluate your medicine list and assess whether alcohol or another substance is compounding your memory loss. Usually, after teasing out all these factors, a skilled professional will be able to determine if part of your memory problem is really, truly Alzheimer's disease, mild cognitive impairment, or some other brain disorder.

Is It My Mood or My Memory?

Don't fall into the trap where people are going to say you're just depressed and you don't have a memory problem—it's "all in your head." Depression in itself, if untreated, increases your risk for losing your memory, either from small strokes in your brain or from Alzheimer's disease or another form of dementia. If you are in the midst of grief, from the loss of a partner, or a parent, or a child leaving home, the dramatic change in neurotransmitters in your brain and body may set the scene for brain fog and a sense of memory loss that's similar to Alzheimer's disease but is *not* Alzheimer's disease (section I of this clinic). In addition, severe trauma such as physical, emotional, or sexual abuse or post-traumatic stress disorder releases cortisol, which equally "gums up" the memory apparatus in the hippocampus (section II). However, by aggressively treating the disorders addressed in those cases, mood, irritability, anxiety, and trauma, you are reducing your risk for dementia.

Brain Changes Associated with Memory Problems

When it comes to understanding the treatments for memory problems, it's important to understand the brain changes associated with diseases that cause memory loss. When we experience normal aging, which, I might add, is not a disease, memory changes from our earlier life. The most obvious difference is that we may retrieve memory at a slower rate. The mildest memory disorder, or perhaps memory disease, is mild cognitive impairment. And then people describe Alzheimer's disease in terms of a range of severity: early, moderate, and severe. Perhaps by the time you're reading this book, the names will be different. Brain science as a field is rapidly changing. To diagnose memory problems, physicians and scientists are looking at proteins that can be found in a brain that has Alzheimer's or other memory disorders.

In Alzheimer's disease, scientists are currently looking at a protein—amyloid-beta precursor protein—that affects learning and memory. Scientists are looking for forms of amyloid protein in the blood and brain fluid to see if they can detect increased levels in people who have early stages of Alzheimer's disease. Similarly, scans are being developed to show if we, the potential patient, may have abnormal amounts of this protein built up in our brain and whether or not those levels are somehow related to memory symptoms, indicating the presence of Alzheimer's disease, chronic traumatic encephalopathy, brain injury, or some other memory disorder.[25]

However, an important note: though these tests may be performed on an experimental basis in several major medical centers, the same physicians who are designing the tests have a big problem. What is it? They are trying to create a diagnostic test to determine if you have Alzheimer's disease, but they don't know what to do or how to treat you if they find you do. Western medicine doesn't have a potent treatment to treat Alzheimer's disease if a test were to prove you have it. So should you have the test? Some physicians and scientists say that if you were to get a positive result, it would help you with the planning of your life. *Ehh . . .* Other scientists and physicians suggest that by working with these proteins and scans, it may help them down the road devise treatments directed against those purported proteins that seem to be at the scene of the crime, near the "injury" in the brains of Alzheimer's patients.

You don't need to have one of these scans to find out that you may have a progressive illness of memory. After getting a neuropsychological assessment for learning and memory, an MRI, and perhaps blood tests to rule out reversible causes of memory loss, you'll be able to elucidate to what degree you may have a deterioration of the networks in your brain, memory or otherwise. Consider the solutions below. But I don't know if I would want someone, with one of these scans, with data that they're only in the early stages of understanding, to tell me what my future is going to be like. And though someone may argue that it's important to plan one's future, how can one really know what the future is? The course of any illness, such as cancer, lupus, chronic fatigue, Lyme, or even Alzheimer's disease or mild cognitive changes, is different for one person than for another, depending on their diet, their treatment for depression, their capacity for exercise, or changes in how they conduct their lives.

So I'm not going to describe in this book what happens to a person when they're "mild, or moderately, or severely impaired" with this disorder and what the "usual course" is. Suffice it to say that in the milder forms of Alzheimer's disease, you may be able to conduct your life as usual with more support from your friends and family, but in the more severe forms, you will have trouble dressing and taking care of yourself and need a lot more support. In the milder forms, you may forget names, misplace items, not remember recent events, but people—secretaries, spouses—will be able to cue or remind you. However, in the more severe forms, it will become essential that others run your financial and day-to-day physical care. It's your mind, and with the help and support of your treatment team, the physicians, acupuncturists, naturopaths, cognitive behavioral therapists, spiritual counselors, family, and loved ones, you're going to create wholeness and revive to the best of your ability the circuits in your brain.

After Your Tests

What's the point of getting all these tests? As of this writing, Western medicine, as I've said, has very limited options for medicines to treat mild cognitive impairment versus mild to moderate to severe Alzheimer's disease. Currently available drugs like Aricept and others may at best show some improvement in daily function, but they don't appear to slow the course of the illness. On the other hand, there are other treatments that do seem to lessen its impact or progression.

The best treatments for memory disorders that involve dementia are ones that impact inflammation and cardiovascular disease. Science shows us that many of the risk factors for Alzheimer's disease are the same ones that involve cardiovascular disease. For example, APOE4 is a risk factor for both cholesterol problems and Alzheimer's disease. Namenda is a medicine that decreases inflammation and may help with the early to moderate stages of Alzheimer's disease. In addition, coenzyme Q10, alpha-tocotrienol, and other high-potency anti-inflammatories may help with the inflammatory basis behind degenerative memory problems.[26]

THE SOLUTION

In addition to the suggestions above, consider the following steps to improve your brain circuits.

Reduce stress and cortisol. Many of the long-term stressors in our lives help accelerate the onset of memory loss as well as the progression of memory degenerative disorder. If you've had a loss of a loved one, or the "empty house syndrome," you want to fill your house and your life with loved ones. If you can't find them, create them. Go to your nearest spiritual centers or recreational centers, volunteer, create "prosthetic" family members when your own have left this world. The stress of untreated grief enhances long-term changes in the hippocampus and other areas of the brain that may disrupt memory function.

Grow memory circuits. If you want to increase your capacity for memory, you want to promote lifelong learning and change, so you need to add mental, emotional, and social stimulation to your life. Yes, any amount of change and new learning is to some degree stressful, so if you have problems with social anxiety, phobia, grief, or sadness, go to your nearest mental health center and get someone who knows cognitive behavioral therapy or supportive therapy to help you handle the emotional and social factors that complicate memory loss.[27]

Use medical intuition to improve your memory. On a piece of paper, draw seven circles, one above the other. Label those centers 1 through 7 from the bottom up. From a medical intuitive point of view, we have seven centers in our life. When we have an accumulation of losses in our lives, these centers start to empty out. So on your diagram, write the number 14 percent next to each one. Why? Because if you have a loss in any area of your life, you've lost one-seventh of your life, or 14 percent. So, for example, if you've lost loved ones, a partner, a husband, or a wife, you've just lost 14 percent in your second center. Have you retired? You just lost your third center, another 14 percent. Has your family moved away? Have other family members died? First center—yet another 14 percent. So let's add that up: 42 percent of your life has, in essence, died. That's almost half of your life that has left, creating a gaping hole, a sense of emptiness.

Center by center, use medical intuition to take account of all the losses or vacancies in your life. These are the centers you now have to reconstitute by transplanting new people and experiences into your life. In this way you'll also begin to reconstitute your mind-body health, not to mention your memory. By adding or transplanting groups of people who are in a way families (first center), you add nutrients of belonging to support your brain chemistry away from depression and anxiety. By having some kind of avocation, work, or purpose that challenges your mind and body (third center), you release opiates and dopamine, neurochemicals of reward that may keep your learning and memory centers operational. And finally, being open to the possibility of a relationship after a lost love (second center), or even surrounding yourself with buddies and friends, provides you social support, freedom from anxiety, that may help buffer cortisol levels in your brain and further protect your memory machinery. And while you're at it, have a trusted advisor, counselor, or family member help you determine if there's any residual sadness, panic, or trauma from these losses that may also impact your memory.

OTHER REMEDIES

Please go to the other sections in this chapter on how to build your memory by learning how to reduce inflammation and promote the production of acetylcholine, GABA, serotonin, norepinephrine, dopamine, and other neurotransmitters. Consider following all the other suggestions to improve your memory, whether it's acupuncture, hyperbaric oxygen, or evaluating your med list to see if there may be deleterious substances that are gumming up your brain circuits. All of these suggestions may promote improvement of memory.

Consider getting a pet or a plant that you need to take care of every day. Studies suggest that even patients with moderate dementia in nursing homes have improved memory scores when they have to take care of something living. In addition to supplements like acetyl-L-carnitine, CPD-choline, vitamin E, DHA, folic acid, B6, and B12, Siberian ginseng, ginkgo biloba, and zinc, you might want to consider huperzine-A 60 to 200 micrograms per day. This Chinese moss may raise acetylcholine activity and has been shown to improve memory in Alzheimer's disease, normal aging, and multi-infarct dementia. Similar to donepezil, this supplement may increase memory neural network efficiency and help prevent nerve cell death. Natural forms of this substance may be three to four times more potent than synthetic forms. (For dosages of all these supplements and herbs, go to the previous cases in this clinic.)

The Affirmations

We're all concerned to some degree about maintaining a healthy mind and memory, not to mention a healthy body, as we age. Louise asks you to evaluate the following list of thoughts.

- Growing old frightens me.
- What if I have a painful death?
- I'll never be able to face old age.
- Everyone in my family seems to get dementia. It's hopeless.
- I'm afraid of the future.
- I'm no longer wanted.
- There's no support left in my life.
- I need to control everything around me.
- I give up.

Louise offers a variety of affirmations to help us change a mind-set that can fossilize our brain circuits and make it hard for us to have healthy memory throughout our life.

- For memory, divine protection, safety, peace: "The intelligence of the Universe operates at every level of my life."

- For aging: "I love and accept myself at every age, at every moment of my life."

- For Alzheimer's disease in particular, which is a refusal to deal with the world as it is, hopelessness, helplessness, and anger: "There is always a new and better way to see and experience life. I forgive and release the past and move into joy."

- For the thought pattern "I'm afraid of getting old": "Every age has its infinite possibilities. My age is perfect and I enjoy each new moment."

- If you are suffering from memory symptoms or difficulty operating your brain efficiently and effectively in your life right now after using all the solutions in this chapter: "I trust the process of life. I am on an endless journey through eternity."

- When it comes to accessing all of our potential in our mind for memory, consider this affirmation: "The point of power is always in the present moment."

Chapter 6

BODY, MIND, BRAIN

Much of my career as a medical intuitive and neuropsychiatrist is spent uncovering the ways in which certain emotions are associated with physical illnesses. What I have found, ironically, especially as a psychiatrist, is that often someone will come to a doctor feeling anxious and depressed for the first time in their life and there seems to be no reason why they're feeling that emotion. They're not worried about their family, relationship, or work, and they don't seem to have grief about the death of a loved one, a failed marriage, or the loss of a job. And then, after a physical exam and some basic tests, we find out that they have a health problem in their body. That anxiety, irritability, sadness, was the first and only symptom that alerted anyone to the presence of a serious health problem, whether it was an autoimmune problem, hormonal imbalance such as thyroid insufficiency, adrenal gland abnormality, estrogen, testosterone, or other hormonal problems. Brain fog, moodiness, and memory problems may have been the first warning signs that they had a serious digestive problem, cardiac or lung problem, brain disorder, or even cancer of some kind.

Everyone has heard these kinds of scenarios:

- A person is anxious, tired, nervous, and just a little achy and has problems paying attention after years of feeling more or less normal. The person goes to the doctor and gets treated for depression. The medicine or nutritional supplements don't work. Finally someone runs tests and the person is diagnosed with lupus.

- A man feels sad, insecure about a recent failed marriage and bankruptcy. He's irritable and moody, feels guilty, and is constantly apologizing. He goes to the doctor and gets treated for depression with nutritional supplements, herbs, and medicines. They don't work, and he still feels depressed, guilty, sad, and weak. Someone checks his testosterone levels and finds out they're very low. After replacement of his testosterone, though he's still sad about his bankruptcy and failed marriage and is "working it through" in therapy, he's in a better place to handle his thoughts and reconstitute his life.

- We feel nervous and edgy and have more and more problems focusing and paying attention at work. Because we are in our 50s, we think it's just changes in estrogen and progesterone. So we get treatment for the moodiness and irritability that accompany "the change." However, after eight months we still feel uneasy, tense, and panicky, and our brain is in a daze. A gastroenterologist tests us for bacterial overgrowth in our small intestine as well as celiac disease and finds out we have both disorders. After going on a special diet and reducing the buildup of endotoxins in our gut (and throughout our system, including the blood), we become calm, collected, and focused.

- Someone goes to the emergency room with nervousness out of the blue when they've never had panic attacks before in their life. They're discharged.

Four hours later they go back to the emergency room with the same amount of panic, and an astute doctor orders a scan on their lungs and finds out they have clots—a condition called a pulmonary embolism.

- A woman gets anxiety, feels stressed, with "butterflies in her stomach." She goes to a doctor who sends her to the emergency room, and after an EKG and cursory tests, which are negative, she is told that it's just stress and anxiety. The scenario is repeated on three consecutive weekends, and though the woman has never had an abnormal EKG, an astute nurse tests her heart enzymes to look for a more serious heart ailment. The results come back positive and show that she's having a heart attack.

- You are nervous, anxious, and depressed in your sophomore year at college, and you have trouble paying attention in your classes. It feels like there's a lump in your throat and your heart is racing just a little bit. You go to the health center and they say you're stressed about school. You take a semester off, with the same symptoms, and your parents get you treatment for panic disorder. In some scenarios you may even drop out of school completely, thinking that you just can't handle it because your panic is so severe. A decade or two will go by and you'll have a variety of vague symptoms, including tense muscles, heart racing, problems paying attention, and of course the panic, all of which you'll treat with medicines, nutritional supplements, herbs, and so on. No one will really think there's anything wrong with your health until you're 35 and you fracture your wrist, develop osteoporosis, and begin to lose your teeth. An astute health care practitioner finds out that you've had a parathyroid disorder for decades and that all your symptoms can be accounted for

HEAL YOUR MIND

by calcium problems, including the emotional and
physical symptoms of panic, not to mention the
fracture and the loss of your teeth.

- Last but not least, you're getting ready to go on a
  Caribbean cruise with your partner and you start to
  feel nervous. You go to your G.P. and they notice you
  have a bit of a respiratory issue. They think you just
  need rest and it might be your asthma kicking up:
  "Just take your inhaler on the ship, relax, and you'll
  be fine." So you go on the cruise, feeling tired and
  still nervous no matter how much you rest. Then on
  the way home you develop clots in your legs (deep
  vein thrombosis, DVT). You go to the emergency
  room and they find out you have lung cancer.

In each of these cases, the first symptom of physical illness
was an emotion.

APPLYING MIND–BODY MEDICINE

Much has been written in the last three or four decades on
mind-body medicine. People are always talking about how their
mind affects their body—the so-called mind over matter. In this
chapter, we're going to talk about how body affects mind. How
your body, through illness, may be the precipitant of a mood, anxiety, irritability, anger, attention, or memory problem. Theoretically, we would think this concept that we're talking about—the
mind can affect the body, the body can affect the mind—would
be easy to comprehend and ultimately utilize to create health. Not
so much. Why? For one, when you explain to people that depression, anxiety, irritability, or anger, when held for a long time, can
increase their chance toward health problems, people feel blamed.
And when people have health problems that are made worse by the
changes in the neurotransmitters associated with mood problems,
like serotonin, epinephrine, GABA, and opiates, they feel blamed
again. Or, worse yet, when you tell someone—or when I myself

am told—that the pain, the headaches, the IBS, seizures, whatever the health problem is, can be made worse by the anxiety or depression, you really hear, "You're telling me it's all in my head." And you'll tend not to want to go to that practitioner anymore.

And when it comes to this chapter, body-mind medicine, why is it equally hard to comprehend and ultimately use? Because when we present with a pure symptom like anxiety or depression or irritability or anger, the majority of professionals are likely to think that the symptom is purely in our head and probably not generated by a health problem in our body.

The title of this book is *Heal Your Mind: Your Prescription for Wholeness through Medicine, Affirmations, and Intuition.* If the mind is made up of one's brain and body, then health problems occur simultaneously in both. It's easy to say, "Is it in my head or is it in my body? Is this structural or is it emotional? Is this depression or is this Lyme? Is this anxiety or is this mercury poisoning? Is this anger or is this heart disease? Is this grief and sadness or a precancerous condition?" We must see that it's neither one nor the other. Both conditions occur simultaneously.

WAYS OF LOOKING AT BODY, MIND, AND BRAIN

I have been in the field of medical intuition for over 30 years. After I outline the emotional issues in someone's life that I see aggravate their health, and then illuminate the symptoms in their body that are causing them "dis-ease," more often than not people say to me, "Dr. Mona Lisa, you don't understand. My problem isn't in my head, it's in my body." I say, "I know, it's both. It's because your head is part of your body."

In this chapter you are going to learn to heal in two major ways. Using medical intuition, you will learn how certain emotional patterns are associated with certain physical symptoms in the body. And when it comes to healing the mind, you will learn to create wholeness by treating both the brain and the body, by learning that the brain may be the first sign that a major illness is beginning to brew in the body.

So if you've had new or even chronic depression, irritability, moodiness, anxiety, and problems with attention, brain fog memory, and addiction, this is the chapter for you. You may just get the key to some additional solutions for finding peace and using your potential.

Louise Hay's first book, *Heal Your Body*, lays out the mental causes for physical illnesses and the metaphysical ways to overcome them. Note that Louise never makes a distinction between brain and body. Despite the book's title, among the listed disorders, ailments of the brain are never listed separately from ailments of the body. Allergies are listed alongside Alzheimer's. You'll see amnesia next to anemia. To think that fear, anger, sadness, and deficiency in love and joy are somehow separate from anemia, Alzheimer's, pain, and suffering seems pretty reasonable. Back then in the '70s, she equated body and mind, brain and body, physical health and emotional health. It's taken us 40 years to catch up. Maybe we're still trying to.

According to Louise, if you have a health problem, it's considered an excess of fear, anger, or sadness, or a deficiency in love and joy, and this can be changed with a new thought pattern. For example, say you have a problem with depression. According to Louise, the thought pattern behind this is apathy—a resistance to feeling, a deadening of self, and fear. So you change that thought pattern to "It is safe to feel. I open myself to life. I am willing to experience life." In a way, what Louise is doing to change the thought patterns in depression is very similar to what we do in cognitive behavioral therapy in psychiatry today.

She addresses a body problem in the same way. We simply look at the thought pattern, find the affirmation, and change our reasoning. For example, cardiovascular disease. Louise says cardiovascular disease has to do with difficulty carrying the joy of life, a deficiency in joy. So, to lessen your tendency toward that, you would change the thought pattern by doing the affirmation "I am filled with joy. It flows with me in every beat of my heart." And so on.

According to Louise, whether there's a problem in the mind or the body, the therapeutic solution is the same. You find the unhealthy thought pattern, the excess or deficient emotion. You change the thought. You add the emotion that's missing—usually joy and love—and you move on to health. If you were a sophisticated scientist who'd spent years in brain science, neuroanatomy, or had done a psychiatric residency, or accumulated, say, $275,000 in student loans (who might that be?), you might think that that was simplistic and whistle in offense. You might even say to yourself, "The audacity of this woman, to think that such a simple method could work!" However, then during your training in psychiatry (if you've figured it out, this is me), you would find that the father of cognitive behavioral therapy, Aaron Beck, devised treatment plans to change people's thoughts, and this is the basis behind how cognitive behavioral therapy is done in psychiatry today. The protocols, or "recipes," of cognitive behavioral therapy are similar statements—though more convoluted—to the ones Louise Hay uses in her slim book. Statements to treat anxiety, depression, anger. And we know now in the 21st century that many of those emotions, if sustained, increase our chance toward a variety of unrelenting health problems such as heart disease, cancers, dementia, diabetes, obesity, chronic pain, immune system disorders, and the like.[1]

THE SCIENCE OF MEDICAL INTUITION: HOW EMOTIONS BECOME HEALTH PROBLEMS AND HEALTH PROBLEMS BECOME EMOTIONS

Emotions register as symptoms in your body, and the beginning of illness in your body may be first noticed only as an emotion like fear, anger, sadness, or brain fog. In Chapter 1, we talked about an emotion-disease domino effect in which, if an emotion or a mood is held for very long, it sets off cascades of inflammatory mediators. If you feel long-term depression, anxiety, panic, or sadness, the mood gets transferred to your brain stem or your adrenal gland, epinephrine and cortisol are released, then inflammatory mediators like cytokines and others cause a domino effect of changes in your body. Fever, weakness, lethargy, then a virus or allergy, then over time hormonal changes, arthritis, cholesterol, insulin, blood pressure, and weight problems, addiction, and other body problems spiral out of control.

Similarly, if you have a health problem in your body, there is a disease-mood domino effect. Whether it's an overgrowth in bacteria in your bowel with a release of inflammation molecules, endotoxins, that leak into your blood and then travel into your brain, making you feel depressed, anxious or irritable; or inflammatory mediators, such as TNF-alpha and others, of rheumatoid arthritis and other autoimmune disorders leaking out from your achy joints into your blood system, into your brain, causing you to feel lethargic, weepy, tearful, irritable, edgy, and snappy. You may not even know you're having another "flare-up" of your autoimmune problem until you get in an argument out of the blue with a loved one over nothing, really. Then you realize that you're sick again and that the only sign to you that your joint problem is going south is that switch in your mood.

And finally, you may be in remission for your lung cancer, sailing through life with utter relief, when out of the blue you feel depressed. Even though you are tearful and have brain fog, you take a fearless inventory of your life to find out what might be depressing you—and you don't find anything. Only to go to your next checkup and have your doctor find out that you have a tiny tumor in your lung. Your doctor says you have a disorder that comes along with cancer called a paraneoplastic syndrome that releases chemicals from your lung into your blood that travel to your brain and make you feel depressed and act loopy. In all of these cases in which there is a body-brain domino effect, mood, anxiety, irritability, and attention problems were only the first symptom that intuitively pointed out to you that something was up in your body.[2]

In this chapter, Louise and I want to help you truly create wholeness in your mind. To really heal our mind and create wholeness, we need to heal the brain and the body simultaneously. Healing the mind, in fact, is understanding that body and mind are merely parts of one whole being.

So if you have had short-term or even long-term depression, irritability, moodiness, or anxiety problems, not to mention short- or long-term health problems, step into the All Is Well Clinic. By addressing those aspects in your body that may also be affecting your mood, sense of peace, and capacity to use all of your intellect, you will be on your path to total healing.

THE ALL IS WELL CLINIC

If you want to know another way of solving your depression, panic, attention, addiction, learning, and memory problems, these case studies ahead are for you. We're going to look to the body to find out what health problems may be making your mind disorder worse. Whether you have immune system problems or a hormonal, digestive, weight, cardiovascular, or other disorder, there's always some element of a health problem in our body below our neck that's affecting the function of our brain.

I. IMMUNE DISORDERS, ADRENAL GLAND FUNCTION, AND THE BRAIN

Have you been concerned about your immune system, whether it's allergy, autoimmune problems, or infections? Have you been concerned about adrenal gland function, whether it's fatigue, weight gain, or other problems? Ask yourself if you have the following symptoms:

- You've been diagnosed with fibromyalgia or chronic fatigue or some other virus or bacterial infection such as Lyme disease or others.

- You have allergies that influence your skin, digestion, and respiratory tract, to name but a few.

- You've been diagnosed with a variety of autoimmune disorders like lupus, rheumatoid arthritis, psoriasis, Hashimoto's, Graves' disease, or others.

- You have fatigue or infections.
- You have weight gain in the central part of your body.
- You have moodiness or irritability.
- You have striae, lines in your skin.
- You easily bruise.
- You have a host of peculiar symptoms of fatigue, joint achiness, and vague physical complaints that are hard to describe.

If you have anxiety, depression, irritability, brain fog, and problems with your memory in addition to many of the above symptoms, consider the following reading.

Abigail: Paralyzed by Anxiety

Abigail, 37, called me for a reading. She was having problems with new depression and paralyzing anxiety.

The Intuitive Reading

Abigail appeared to be in one of those dead-end relationships. She seemed to pick the wrong man over and over again. A man who wasn't there for her. Worse yet, the men she picked cheated on her. Abigail's brain and body seemed to have a backlog of depression from a series of failed relationships. However, she also seemed to have the nervousness, the anxiety, and the jitters of someone who is waiting for the next tragedy to happen in her life.

The Body

I noticed problems with focus, attention, and brain fog. However, the most significant aspect of Abigail's body to me was that her immune system seemed to be "on fire." Was this her immune system's capacity to make antibodies against several organs? I saw red dots on her joints, skin, thyroid, and bowel. And did Abigail have problems with her fertility, making it hard for her to have children? Her hormones seemed to go up and down, up and down, and that seemed to parallel her moods.

THE FACTS

Abigail told me that the doctors had picked up antibodies in her blood for lupus and Addison's disease (low adrenal gland function). She had diffuse joint pain as well as multiple medical problems from both autoimmune disorders. In addition to the joint pain, kidney, thyroid, and low cortisol levels she had from both these autoimmune problems, Abigail suffered from anxiety and depression that no medicine could treat. She wanted to know, was it her hormones? Estrogen and progesterone? Were Abigail's anxiety and depression symptoms generated from her brain in response to a series of failed relationships and lifelong trauma? Or were her anxiety and depression due to her lupus and Addison's disease, the inflammation from her low cortisol, and inflammation from autoimmune attack on her joints, kidneys, and hormonal organs? The answer is both. In order for Abigail to heal, she had to create a prescription that addressed her whole being, both her brain's and her body's symptoms.

Let's first address the adrenal gland, mood, and anxiety.

ADRENAL GLAND AND MOOD

If you have the deficient cortisol of Addison's disease or the excess cortisol of Cushing's syndrome, either extreme can increase your chance toward anxiety, depression, and brain fog. It seems ironic that too much and too little of the same hormone can both cause depression and anxiety, but it's true. And, while we're at it, the same can be true for other hormones as well, including estrogen, thyroid, and others. Specifically estrogen: estrogen excess, either from excess body fat stores or from hormone replacement, is notorious for causing depression. Too little estrogen, especially the sudden change of hormone levels in menopause and postpartum, can cause depression too. So it seems that too little or too much

251

of any hormone in our body can disrupt the intricate emotional circuitry in our brain's limbic system.

But there's more. Every single day, hormones are released in our brain and body according to a circadian rhythm. All of our hormones are keyed in to the ups and downs of cortisol. That means the adrenal gland is in charge, in a way, of all your other hormones. The normal rhythm is for cortisol to be high in the morning and low at night. If you have the reverse pattern—low levels of cortisol in the morning and high levels at night—you're more likely to have depression. So if you're just testing your cortisol levels at one time of the day versus the other, that's not going to help you. In the end, we want balance; we want to establish a normal rhythm, an ebb and flow of hormones in our brain and body throughout the whole day.

But let's move on to the immune system and mood.

Immune System Disorders and Mood

There are many areas in our emotional brain that biochemically act in the same way as our immune system. What does that mean? It means that when our immune system gets fired up, whether through infection, allergy, or autoimmune problems, it may affect our mood. If we were to get lupus, rheumatoid arthritis, a chronic infection like Lyme, chronic fatigue, or fibromyalgia, food allergy, psoriasis, or eczema, the inflammation in our body would be more likely to irritate our mood, increasing our chance toward depression, anxiety, brain fog, memory problems, maybe even addiction. So understand, if you are being treated for any or all of these disorders, we have to follow the title of that famous book by Joan Borysenko: we need to simultaneously mind the body and mend the mind.

Cortisol has a tremendous impact on our immune system. On the one hand, doctors give us steroids, a form of cortisol, to lower the inflammation in autoimmune disorders like rheumatoid arthritis, lupus, psoriasis, and others. You may, even now, be using "glandulars" or other ways of supplementing adrenal gland cortisol "naturally." On the other hand, when we are anxious, panicky, or depressed, those hormones can get transmitted to our adrenal gland, causing the adrenal gland to release unhealthy levels of cortisol. Those "stress"-related changes in our adrenal gland cortisol release can ironically elicit an infection, an allergy, an autoimmune illness, or something more serious. (See the other sections in this chapter.) But chances are if you have adrenal gland problems, you have immune system problems. If you have immune system problems, you have adrenal gland problems. And ultimately, if you have adrenal gland *and* immune system problems, you're also more likely to have depression, anxiety, irritability, and problems with focus and memory, not to mention addiction.

So whether you have adrenal gland problems or what people are currently calling "adrenal gland fatigue," cortisol either in excess or in deficiency is likely to cause you depression, anxiety, and panic. If you have a chronic infection like Lyme, Epstein-Barr virus, fibromyalgia, chronic allergies, environmental illness, you aren't just prone to pain, fatigue, and sleepiness. You're also more likely to have problems with depression, anxiety, brain fog, inattention, and memory. But there's hope. If we treat both brain and body simultaneously, both mood and immunity, pain and panic, attention and agony, emotional and physical madness may improve.

THE MEDICAL INTUITIVE SOLUTION

What is the solution? How do you support the brain and the body simultaneously?

First, do a medical intuitive reading on your life. What is your body telling you about what in your life, or in the life of a loved one, needs to change? Start your medical intuitive reading in the following way. Draw a large box and label it BODY. In the box, draw seven circles, one above the other. Label them 1 through 7 from the bottom up. Where in your body is the immune system giving you symptoms?

Refer to the chart of energy centers in Appendix A. You'll see that on the right side the organs of the body are listed alongside the corresponding centers. Put an X on the regions where you have immune system problems. Then read the emotional issues on the left side of the chart to find the emotional area that coincides with your health problem. The beginning of your healing is connecting body with mind, the physical symptom with the area in your life that you are emotionally and intuitively needing to examine.

Once you've connected your body symptoms with what your medical intuition is wanting you to focus on in your life, what is the first step? Get a trusted coach, counselor, or other guide to help you take a "fearless inventory" of your reading. Perhaps it may be helpful to bring along a close friend who is, let us just say, extremely honest yet loving and supportive. They may help you find out what the next steps are and what needs to change in the emotional areas you've marked on your medical intuitive reading chart.

Second, support the body. While you're learning how to evaluate and respond to the way medical intuition is speaking to you through your body and brain, you must support your whole body's capacity to heal physically. You can use medicines, nutritional supplements, herbs, and diet to support your immune system. See *All Is Well: Heal Your Body with Medicine, Intuition, and Affirmations*, the first center chapter, for specific suggestions on immune system dysfunction.

The third and final step is to rewire the memory and thoughts that are connected in the network between mind and body, body and mind. Using affirmations, cognitive behavioral therapy, and other body therapies like EMDR, somatic release, and others, we can learn to change the thought patterns about what's going on in our life or our response to the lives of those around us. Using affirmations can change not only how you see your life or the lives of others, but how you see the world, and it can help you follow your intuition and respond to it effectively. Your health problem will ultimately lead you to not just to a healthier mind-set and wisdom; you will, as a result of this crisis, have greater access to your intuition and be able to respond to it more effectively in the future. In the end you will find that you begin to see your unique pattern through which your body-mind is literally letting you know intuitively how to help create wholeness in your life.

II. HORMONES, HEART ISSUES, AND THE BRAIN

Have you had some problems with depression, anxiety, and irritability, but more or less become stable until midlife? Have you started to tinker with your supplements, medicines, and other remedies, but no matter what you do, you can't stabilize your mood? Then you may look to your hormones, your heart, and your cardiovascular system for some clues as to what may make your brain's mood circuits begin to spiral out of control.

Have you hit that stage in your life where your hormones can't possibly get more out of control? Does your heart race? Is your anxiety off the charts? Do you have trouble falling asleep and staying asleep? Is your body keyed up, tense, stomach in a knot? Whether it's high blood pressure, unstable blood pressure, or heart palpitations, many of these cardiac disorders can be subtle, even silent. Here's how subtle the signs can be.

- Again, many people don't even know they are having an arrythmia or even a heart attack, especially women; the only symptoms they may experience are anxiety, breathlessness, and panic. They may not know it until many years later when the scarring on their heart is revealed by way of an abnormal EKG.

- High blood pressure is notorious for being "the silent killer"; those who have been lucky enough to have received the diagnosis and received treatment have mentally learned the subtleties in their brain and body that signal when their "pressure is rising." They may experience the beginnings of restlessness, irritability, and extreme frustration.

- Many a man enters a "midlife crisis" where he gets down in the dumps, lethargic, only to find out that

that extreme depression is signaling plummeting testosterone levels.

- And finally, last but not least, how many women have you heard of (maybe it's you) who've had a hysterectomy or antihormonal treatment for breast cancer and become profoundly depressed? The crying, the tearfulness, the extreme plummeting of mood, not to mention the occasional hot-trigger temper, may also occur in a woman who's just delivered her baby. At a time when you're supposed to be in utter bliss, holding a "bundle of joy," you're not feeling so joyful.

Science is only just now tracing those inflammation pathways between our bodies, hormone centers, heart and blood vessels, and our brain's mood regions. The two-way domino effect between brain and body, body and brain, in this section concerns two regions in the body that are intricately related. Just as in the last section the immune system and adrenal gland cortisol were intertwined systems in the body, so are our hormones, our heart, and our blood vessels.[3]

So if you have had long-term depression, moodiness, irritability, and anxiety, not to mention distractibility and memory problems, watch your body's health particularly closely beginning at midlife. Often, your depression may worsen, your panic may escalate, and your irritability may increase, and these may be the first signs that your hormones and your heart and cardiovascular system health may be veering out of control. Consider the following story.

BLANCHE: HORMONAL ANXIETY

Blanche, 49, called me asking, "Why aren't my antianxiety medications working anymore? Maybe it's my hormones, but I can't get them stable. Why?"

THE INTUITIVE READING

When I looked at Blanche's life, I saw that she was in a family where there was someone who ruled with an iron fist. Was this person bossy? Controlling? Whatever it was, this person controlled money, property, and made people feel guilty. I could just see Blanche bobbing and weaving around this king-like person as the person made angry demands. And if Blanche at all got frustrated, she kept it all inside, not complaining, because she just knew that would make everything worse.

THE BODY

When I intuitively looked into Blanche's body, her head seemed to spin and she had an imbalanced feeling in her body as well. I could see her blood vessels open and close erratically, making her blood pressure swing erratically as well. When it came to her heart, her heart rate was racing all over the place in an irregular rhythm. When I got to her kidneys, it seemed that their arteries were clogged with some white substance. I wondered, could she have trouble with storing fats in her body? The blood vessels in her body seemed frazzled.

Overall, Blanche's whole body felt nervous, keyed up, overwhelmed, tearful, and irritable. However, she tried to keep all of her feelings inside behind a brave and stoic face, and all those keyed-up feelings made it hard for her to fall asleep.

THE FACTS

Blanche said she had suffered from panic for years but had managed to more or less control it with 5-HTP, passion flower, and lemon balm, not to mention cognitive behavioral therapy and affirmations. Frantically, she cried, "But those things aren't working anymore!" Panic-stricken, Blanche had gone to a practitioner who had tried to stabilize her hormones. Progesterone, estrogen, DHEA, pregnenolone . . . the list trailed on. She said, "No matter what I do, I can't get them stable."

Blanche added that she was on an antihypertensive medicine for high blood pressure and she also took meds for her cholesterol. And that bossy member of her family? Oh, that person was her mother, who really made Blanche's blood pressure hit the roof. Not a queen, but a king who ruled with an iron fist. Blanche's mother manipulated her whole family with guilt and coercion. When the phone began to ring, Blanche's blood pressure went up (which she tested on her home blood pressure cuff), and she just knew it was going to be another one of those days of demands. And her weight went up too, along with her cholesterol levels.

THE SOLUTION

If you've had a lifelong struggle with depression, anxiety, irritability, attention, or memory problems, many of the problems in this book, you may have learned to find a variety of prescriptions, whether it's nutritional supplements, medicines, herbs, cognitive behavioral therapy, or affirmations for relief. However, once you hit midlife, your depression, anxiety, irritability, and other brain symptoms may begin to veer out of control again. Why? If you have a variation in some area of your brain, a weakness of sorts, a "barometric change" of hormones at midlife may strain the delicate balance of health you've worked so hard to achieve. With all the intensive changes you've created, whether it's diet, exercise, specific herbal or nutritional supplements, maybe even medicines, when you enter into menopause, or, in men, testopause, you may have to tinker with the doses of what you're taking or try a completely different set of prescriptions. You might not even know that you were entering into the menopause or testopause changes in estrogen, progesterone, and testosterone if it weren't for the changes in your depression, anxiety, irritability, attention, and memory.

If you've been on 5-HTP, that is, a serotonin supplement, or Wellbutrin, a dopamine and norepinephrine medicine, why might these not be enough to maintain your mood? When your estrogen drops, you also lose a hefty dose of its neurotransmitters, dopamine, norepinephrine, and serotonin. Your brain needed those hormones as antidepressant and antianxiety medicine before. So when your dose of estrogen (serotonin, norepinephrine, and dopamine) goes down, you're going to need more supplementation for whatever you're taking. The same is true for testosterone. And when it comes to supplements like passion flower and lemon balm or medicines like Klonopin and Xanax, or even drinking alcohol, those substances and/or medicines provide GABA—so when your progesterone levels start to go down, you're losing GABA, and even if your anxiety was in check before with passion flower, lemon balm, Klonopin, Xanax, or the occasional glass of wine, after menopause the drop in progesterone, with its drop in GABA, makes your anxiety and panic spiral out of control. Not only might you start to drink more (see Chapter 3), you might find that you build up tolerance to the dose of Klonopin and Xanax you're using. Your anxiety and depression both begin to spiral out of control. Both mood symptoms may be the first sign heralding that your hormones are beginning to change.

YOUR MEDICAL INTUITIVE READING

First, do your medical intuitive reading. Draw a large box and label it BODY. In the box, draw seven circles, one above the other. Label them 1 through 7 from the bottom up. Now put an X on the second center and the fourth center. The second center has to do with hormones and reproductive organs and the fourth center has to do with cardiovascular and heart problems.

Refer to the chart of energy centers in Appendix A. On the right side, the organs of the body are listed alongside the corresponding centers. Move to the left side of the chart and you'll find the emotional issues that may correlate with the symptoms in your body. Understand that illness is always in part due to diet, the environment, genetics, and so on, but every illness has an emotional, intuitive component, and in this part of your healing, we are addressing the intuitive aspect of your health and its solution. So, when hormones in particular dovetail with mood, irritability, and anxiety to cause you pain and suffering, we need to take a fearless inventory of what crises and problems may be asking to be addressed in your relationships or finances.

Similarly, when it comes to having problems with cholesterol, hypertension, chest pain, and other heart and blood vessel problems (fourth center), with their attendant moodiness, irritability, and panic, we may be being asked to examine all the partnerships in our life. What are our relationships with our children? Our mothers? If we are stuffing emotion and frustration into our body, it may get tucked into our cardiovascular system, and if we have enduring patterns in how we express emotions in the partnerships in our life, over decades they may increase our chance toward cardiovascular disease. Ironically, the first time we actually may become just a little bit more emotional, irritable, and unhinged is when we start to get hypertension and cardiac problems. So work with a cognitive behavioral therapist, coach, or trusted advisor on the emotional areas in your life that need to be addressed to create health in your body, specifically your cardiovascular system and hormones in this case, as well as to have long-term healthy moods and brain function.

Second, if you're wondering whether you really are going into menopause, or if you're a man, testopause, go to a licensed practitioner and get a hormonal panel of tests. Understand that hormone replacement, in women and men, for the rest of one's life is controversial. If you do get hormone replacement, you may want to consider looking at bioidentical hormones, but be careful with the amount of replacement. If you replace your hormones to the levels of a 20- or 30-year-old, you may be making a huge mistake. Hormones are growth factors. As our bodies get older, they accumulate more genetic injury, toxins, and so on, and there may be an evolutionary advantage to menopause: by removal of estrogen and progesterone we may be protecting our brain, our breasts, our ovaries, and our uterine lining from its growth hormone effects. Some recent studies suggest that the safest time to take hormone replacement is only a couple of years after menopause. Beyond that, some physicians and scientists believe it may increase your chance toward heart disease, stroke, and breast cancer way beyond its benefits in improving your bone density, memory, or sex life. And how about men? Excessive testosterone replacement has been associated with heart attacks.

Remember that not every symptom that you get in perimenopause and testopause need be treated with hormones. If you have a family history of breast cancer, ovarian cancer, endometrial cancer, or stroke, or if you yourself have had any of these problems, you may want to consider another way of treating your menopausal symptoms. And the same is true if you're a man. If prostate cancer, testicular cancer, or other reproductive cancers, even breast cancer, run in your family or if you yourself have had those disorders, you may want to find another way of managing your mood and memory. There are some wonderful books on the subject: *The Wisdom of Menopause* by Christiane Northrup, M.D., has multiple suggestions on how to handle the brain and the body in menopause. Whether it's with Chinese herbs, nutritional supplements, acupuncture, yoga, meditation, or mindfulness, there are a plethora of solutions to help you handle the decade-long period it takes for you to transcend from one stage of your life to another.

And what about cardiovascular disorders? Go to an extremely skilled cardiovascular center. If you're a woman, you might want to consider going to a cardiovascular diagnostic center that has a branch that specializes in just the treatment and evaluation of women's heart problems. The arteries in a woman's heart are smaller and react different than a man's, and the way one detects heart attack or arrhythmia in women is different from their detection in men. Every woman, once she reaches her 40s, should have a thorough cardiovascular workup, even if she doesn't have depression, anxiety, or any of the standard symptoms of heart problems or blood pressure issues. Get a stress test; they will ask you to get on a treadmill, and they will evaluate whether your blood pressure "decompensates" under the stress of exercise. However, we know that it's not just physical stress that makes a woman's heart vessels spasm, it's emotional stress, having to do with second-center relationships or fourth-center children or parents. So before you start your stress test, put a picture of a partner, child, or parent on the machine so that as they are evaluating your cardiovascular function under stress, you can really elicit stress by looking at those areas in your life that provoke it.

Go to Chapter 5 on memory and look at the solutions for maintaining a healthy brain for memory. Many of the antioxidants, anti-inflammatory supplements, and herbs there will also help you maintain a healthy cardiovascular system. Regularly measure your blood pressure. You may not want to wait until you get that first emotional symptom of irritability, moodiness, and anxiety that's your "tell" that your blood pressure is rising. Aggressively treat your blood pressure, because you don't want it to affect your memory and cloud your focus. In addition to medicines you may take, you might also want to consider going to an acupuncturist, Chinese herbalist, or nutritionist for remedies that have been used for centuries to lower one's blood pressure.

The third solution is to connect mind to body and body to mind. Use affirmations that involve menopause and heart disease (see Appendix B), not to mention hypertension. Use the appropriate affirmations for depression (Chapter 1) and anxiety (Chapter 2) if you had those mood symptoms preceding your hormonal and heart problems. Over time, though it will take some time, you may find that slowly but surely your depression lifts, your anxiety calms, your irritability evaporates, and your blood pressure stabilizes. From time to time you may feel that your hormones get "choppy" again and your blood pressure may rise or you may get that sense of frantic feeling or panic that may signal to you that your body is veering a little out of control and you need to attend to your hormones and your heart, your mood, and your relationships with the people in your life.

III. YOUR BRAIN AND CANCER

Did you find that you were sad and distracted for a few months but didn't quite know why? And then you went for a regular checkup and your doctor found cancer. Have you gone through life with everything seeming to be okay, kind of—the usual ups and downs? But you had this irritability; you couldn't focus; and so you went to your doctor and after looking at your blood tests, they sent you to a specialist because they were concerned about cancer.

If this has happened to you, or you remember it happening to a loved one or a friend, you'll understand and appreciate that often depression, anxiety, irritability, and brain fog may be the only signs we have that there's something wrong, seriously wrong, with our health. You may actually ignore those first warning signs, that emotional funk, the restlessness, thinking you're, you know, just depressed. Maybe you just need to go up on your antidepressant dose, take more 5-HTP or whatever nutritional supplement or medicine you're taking, thinking it's "all in your head." I wouldn't do that if I were you. I would learn to listen to my body and what it might be telling me. Consider the following story.

CHARLES: CANCER ON MY MIND

Charles, 52, called me because he was worried about his future.

THE INTUITIVE READING

When I read Charles, I saw he was worried about how long he was going to live. In fact, I could see for a while he had been living life on autopilot, going through the motions, living life as status quo, each day as it came. However, recently, life wasn't coming to Charles so easily. It seems his career had come to a halt. Had he gotten fired? Laid off? Had the company folded? It seemed that the major focus of Charles's life just went *poof,* and without that sense of purpose in his life, he was lost.

THE BODY

Charles's head felt like a closet whose contents had been completely emptied. No, let me rephrase that. It felt like a house whose contents had been removed precipitously into a U-Haul and moved away. Was he having trouble focusing and paying attention? Did he have trouble with his memory? Not only was he lost in his life, he was getting more and more disconnected from people in general.

Continuing on through his body, my attention intuitively went to his chest area. And though the blood vessels in his body seemed stiff and at the same time fragile, that didn't seem like the biggest problem. I saw a dramatic change in the structure of his lungs and chest. There was a mesh-like pattern where his lungs were supposed to be.

THE FACTS

Charles's wife was on the phone with us during the reading and she mentioned that she was concerned about Charles. He was very different. He seemed depressed, a little irritable, and distracted. And his memory! He was forgetting appointments, forgetting people's names, and had even gotten lost while driving. Recently a physician had found a suspicious spot in Charles's right lung, and a biopsy revealed lung cancer. Since he had never smoked, he didn't understand why he had come down with this life-threatening ailment.

Charles's wife said that ten years earlier, he had lost a job due to "complicated circumstances," and then had tried to become a consultant for another company with "poor results." Now he had again been laid off from his job, and he was devastated. Charles's wife wanted to know if his sadness, irritability, and forgetfulness could merely be depression and grief, not just at the loss of his job but at his cancer diagnosis.

THE SOLUTION

If we've had a major loss in our life, the grief, sadness, and depression can be sustained, weaken our immune system's capacity to protect us against developing cancer. So long-term depression can increase your risk for many immune system problems, not to mention cancer. However, some specific cancer cells produce chemicals, antibodies that distort your mood, attention, memory, and thinking in general. This is called paraneoplastic syndrome, or limbic encephalopathy. Some people may not even know they have cancer except via these first vague symptoms of feeling uncharacteristically moody, irritable, and distracted.[4]

Then, once they find the cancer, treatments like chemotherapy and radiation can affect the white matter in your brain, causing your mind to literally move in slow motion. You may find yourself crying more, and people might think you're reacting to the cancer diagnosis, when really it's the medicine *and* the diagnosis. There's a name for this: "chemo brain." Once you start to develop other side effects, like numbness, tingling, and other vague symptoms, you may realize that it's the medicine.

What's the title of this book? *Heal Your Mind: Your Prescription for Wholeness through Medicine, Affirmations, and Intuition.* What was the title of the last book I wrote with Louise? *All Is Well: Heal Your Body with Medicine, Affirmations, and Intuition.* It is up to you, between you and a practitioner, how you want to heal your body. Do you want to use medicine, herbs, supplements? You choose. Do you want to focus on your mind first? Your body first? You choose. I'd do both at the same time, but that's just me.

YOUR MEDICAL INTUITIVE READING

First, do your medical intuitive reading. Draw a large box and label it BODY. In the box, draw seven circles, one above the other. Label them 1 through 7 from the bottom up. Now put an X in two circles: one, the region where your cancer is, and two, the seventh center, for life-threatening illness. Look to the left side of the chart to examine the emotional, intuitive patterns associated with your specific health problem.

When it comes to cancer in general, as well as all life-threatening illnesses, for that matter, we may not look to our life for the "reason" we got sick, and we don't want to just focus on the fact that we're not ready to die yet. Instead, we may find we need to look for a major life purpose for which we want to live. In partnership with spirit, your soul, or whatever you feel comfortable with, start to think about what you think your life purpose is now and what greater purpose you may be being asked to live for. Go to a trusted coach, spiritual counselor, or even psychotherapist to examine the emotional-intuitive areas that were revealed in your medical intuitive reading.

Second, support the body and the brain. Start by supporting your mood. Talk to your doctor or other practitioner about what may be safe to do to support your depression, anxiety, and irritability. Though you may want to begin to try many of the solutions in this book for depression, irritability, and so on, before using any herbs, supplements, or medicines, talk to the doctor who's treating you for cancer. Drugs, herbs, nutritional supplements, may all interact. Get a second opinion. Don't rely on one person to give you a cancer diagnosis; consider going to a major medical center, even if it's out of state, where they can look at your pathology slides and lab results and see your health problem from a different perspective. Get a piece of paper and write down all the treatments and solutions that you may engage in. Resist the temptation to label something "natural" or "unnatural." Beside each treatment, write the risks of engaging in it and the benefits, short-term and long-term. Then write the risks and benefits of *not* using the treatment. In the end, you are the owner of your body. Doctors, naturopaths, nutritionists, acupuncturists, Reiki masters, qi gong masters, and so on, are all consultants. You have to be the one to choose.

Third, use affirmations. Here, when we connect body to mind and mind to body, we address the thought patterns that may stand in the way of us creating healing and wholeness. Go to Appendix B and look up your specific type of cancer, as well as cancer in general.

But first, understand that we don't cause our illnesses. Even though certain foods we eat, things we smoke, or even thoughts we think may increase our risk for an illness like cancer, we don't create it. So resist the impulse to blame yourself for having caused cancer. It's not true! You didn't cause your cancer. And while you're at it, if some well-meaning friend or family member tries to blame you for your illness, politely extricate yourself from the individual, understanding they are really only trying to help. A thought, a food, a gene—they are only one of many multiple factors that may bring on a cancer or get rid of it. We're not blaming ourselves, but supporting the growth and development of a healthy mindset that's conducive to healing body and mind.

IV. Spiritual Transformation of Brain and Body

I have yet to meet anyone who was a shaman or an intuitive healer or a mystic of sorts who didn't have a lot of emotional and physical health problems. When it comes to the mind, I've found that people who work in the field of intuition, myself included, are some of the moodiest, most anxious, irritable, high-strung, blunt, and passionate individuals I have ever met. I've been told, for example, that I would never win any awards in diplomacy. And how I feel about something is never a mystery, despite the fact that the original "Mona Lisa smile" was quite mysteriously deadpan.

I'm no saint, but I've certainly read about them. Many of the great saints who were medically intuitive—Catherine of Genoa, Teresa of Avila, Catherine de Ricci, and Thérèse of Lisieux among them—were notorious for having "unique minds." They were often eccentric, temperamental, anxious, and very direct and cutting when they delivered their prophetic, intuitive information. And when it comes to their physical health in their body, many intuitive advisors have difficulty. Intuitive advisors often have a variety of hard-to-treat, reactive, complex health problems, including migraine headaches, weight and thyroid problems, and immune system disorders, to name a few.

Suffice it to say that whenever I'm told about someone who they say is a mystic, a shaman, or a medical intuitive, I don't ask for stories illustrating their unique spiritual, intuitive, and mystical gifts. I check out their mind and body. First, the mind: Are they moody? Anxious? Irritable? Cranky? Easy to get in an argument with? Then, the body: How many surgeries have they had? How many times have they almost died? Have they nearly bled to death? Migraine headaches, epilepsy, autoimmune problems, or thyroid disorders?

If the answer is yes to many of these questions, I know these individuals are the real thing. All the shamans and native healers of indigenous tribes, as well as the intuitive healers who came later in history, had a lot of health problems because one's tendency to be intuitively porous, mystically inclined, is related to having a reactive brain and body. So, for those who are mystics, medical intuitives, spiritual advisers and healers, and so on, have to pay close attention to their emotional and physical health, which tends to go down the tubes sometimes.

So, is this you? You may find that you've been "on your spiritual path" for years and along the way you notice changes in your mood, anxiety, memory, not to mention your physical health. Believe me, by being on that path you are leaving ordinary life on earth and wanting to create an extraordinary life by touching the divine. It may take a while for your body and brain to adapt to your new, porous, sensitized, globalized brain-set. Consider the following story.

DENISE: THE MYSTICAL BRAIN

Denise, 37, called me because she was on a spiritual path and she wanted to learn how to straighten her health out so she could access her intuition better.

THE INTUITIVE READING

When I looked at Denise's life, specifically family, oh my God, the chaos! Chaos, chaos everywhere! I could see constant arguments between parents and siblings. If there was someone in the house, there was an argument going on. You could just see Denise hiding behind a door as her parents and other relatives were arguing in the other room. Was she avoiding violence? Was she avoiding being the next target of emotional and physical abuse? It felt like she was one of those little animals in the woods, shaking, hiding underneath a tree, for fear of getting caught by a predator. And then I could see Denise intuitively know when an argument was about to erupt. I could see her standing between the individuals arguing. Was she mediating, brokering peace?

THE BODY

It felt like Denise's body had gone through a war zone. Her brain felt numb, the kind of numbness you feel if you are stuck on an airport runway at JFK, constantly hearing jets overhead. There were pressure headaches, neck pain. Her head felt hot as lightning. I saw a red dotted pattern where her thyroid was supposed to be. Did Denise have problems with chest pressure? There was shortness of breath, nausea, dizziness, vertigo.

When I got to Denise's digestive tract, I could see that she manipulated her health by forever changing her diet. Was this due to food intolerances or allergies? I could see that these nutritional maneuvers helped her for about a month, maybe two months, but eventually any improvement stopped. There seemed to be a lifelong struggle with weight and food restriction too. And finally, I saw sadness, like a blanket, enveloping Denise, with waves of panic that affected her capacity to pay attention and focus in school.

THE FACTS

Denise said she had had problems with her brain and her health since youth, but no one could tell her why. She had always known she was different. Since puberty, she'd fallen a lot, but not really passed out. She was in an automobile accident, but no one was hurt. She was the "black sheep" in the family. People told her she was too sensitive and too emotional.

When it came to school, Denise said she wasn't in the "in" group. She tried to make up for feeling like a social outcast by excelling academically, but that didn't work, either. She studied for tests and quizzes twice and three times as long as everyone else, but she just couldn't get the right answers on tests. Starting in high school, Denise began getting treatment for anxiety and depression. However, after a year of college, she dropped out because she just couldn't keep up with the reading.

Denise told me she just wanted to be normal. She had finished a certificate program in massage therapy, but she said, "I'm just too intuitively connected to the problems of my clients." Recently, she'd had an MRI and other testing to find out why she was having dizziness, vertigo, and chest pain. All the tests were negative. Only one test was slightly abnormal—an EEG showed atypical slow waves. The doctors didn't know how to interpret it.

THE SOLUTION

If you, like Denise, have always felt unique, maybe a black sheep in your family, congratulations! On some level, you don't want to be ordinary, you want to be extraordinary. However, with our unique genius wired in our brain, we somehow need to find happiness and health and lead productive lives.

If you've always had a unique brain that's afforded you learning disabilities and episodes of panic, anxiety, and depression, yes, it's important to love yourself just the way you are. And to love yourself, you need to know how your brain works so you can utilize it in the best way possible. To get a set of operating instructions on how to best work the circuits in your brain for mood, anxiety, learning, attention, and memory, go to a behavioral neurologist or neuropsychology department at a major medical center. They will ask you all about your history: Did you have a history of violence? Brain injury? Abuse? Did you have trouble learning in school? Did you have trouble staying still or focusing? And then they may run a variety of tests, including the one in this case, such as EEGs, MRIs, and so on. Behavioral neurologists, neuropsychiatrists, and neuropsychologists will help you elucidate what is unique about your brain so you can best use it. Don't wait decades to do this. You don't want to miss opportunities in education or career advancement as you experience failure in both. There is a way you can learn how to, with support and instruction, identify what made you different, and with remediation have more successful relationships, finances, and career.[5]

There are a variety of different brain styles that occur in people who are spiritual and mystical. The temporal lobe in our brain specifically is a key area that functions for intuition, spirituality, and mysticism. Whether one has injury there through emotional or physical trauma, epilepsy, or other disorders, one may have exaggerated gifts for spirituality. But all of us have a capacity for mysticism. How? At night when we dream, especially between the hours of 2 and 4 A.M., our hippocampus, yes, that area for memory, has microseizures. These microseizures may be involved not just with memory or dreams, but connecting with the divine.

Saint Paul, Mohammed, Margery of Kempe, Joan of Arc, all had some form of seizures in this temporal lobe region. Joan of Arc had ecstatic states in which she heard the voice of an angel and saw a great light when she had seizures. Catherine of Genoa also had seizures, in which she had hot flashes (does that sound kind of menopausally common for all of us?) as well as sleepwalking and other seizure-like phenomena. Theresa of Avila had visions too; in addition to chronic headaches, she would lose consciousness and also have other seizure symptoms. Catherine de Ricci had complex partial seizures that induced visual hallucinations and mystical states. Emanuel Swedenborg—yep, that guy who started a whole religion—had seizures that involved multiple senses, whether it was smelling, tasting, or feeling things. Joseph Smith had seizures as well. That man who started Mormonism saw a pillar of light and heard voices in episodes where he said he could "look up at heaven." And finally, Ann Lee, who started the Shaker movement, had epilepsy too, with episodes where she would see and hear things.

What does this mean for you? If you're drawn to spirituality, you may be rewiring your temporal lobe, or if your temporal lobe has been rewired by trauma, you may be a savant for intuition. Either way, the fact is you have the brain and the body for intuition and mysticism; however, you may have noticed the fallout in your body, because the temporal lobe has huge amounts of connections to our body, especially our immune system, adrenal glands, hormones, digestive tract, and heart.

So as you are on your spiritual path, or writing down your dreams, or talking with your therapist about your trauma, or you're a full-blown mystic living in an ashram somewhere, you must simultaneously treat the health of both your brain and your body while you are acquiring altered states, mysticism, and intuition.

THE AFFIRMATIONS

If you're a black sheep and you stand out from the rest of the family, you may be sick of being criticized by them. On the other hand, as you move down your spiritual path, you may find there are more and more people whom you don't feel like you belong with, because they don't seem spiritual enough. Consider Louise Hay's premise: *I love myself just the way I am.* As you evolve spiritually, you may also grow to see that even though you may feel different from other people, though they're not also on your spiritual path, we are all still human. And by seeing the similarities in all of us, we can learn to love all of us just the way we are.

MYSTICISM: THE DELICATE BALANCE BETWEEN MIND AND BODY FOR HEALTH

Which leads me to the next set of solutions: radical acceptance. Working with someone who understands dialectical behavioral therapy will help you balance your mystical awareness of other people's problems with knowing when to help. Medical intuitives are notorious for feeling guilty if they don't try to rescue someone whose pain they are intuitively connected to. So work with a cognitive behavioral coach to help you learn skills to balance the emotional mind (right brain) with the rational mind (left brain).

While you're at it, you'll also be able to learn to balance your intuitive, mystical temporal lobe with that more earthbound frontal lobe. You will learn how to operate your evolving brain as you progress on your spiritual and mystical path. Yes, you will *always* be sensitive, but you can and will learn how to gradually become less emotionally and physically reactive to the problems of people around you. And though you may not be able to do much about your intuitive and spiritual porousness that you may have been born with, or may have been a by-product of your trauma or the aftermath of a variety of health problems in your brain and body, DBT and other cognitive behavioral therapies will help you more effectively respond so that your mood, anxiety, distractibility, memory, and health problems come back to a tolerable level that is "normal" for you.

THE WHOLE STORY

Setting aside all the nitty-gritty, the nuts and bolts, and the minutiae of healing your mind, what's the take-home message? What's THE fundamental key point we all need to know to heal?

We have, in this book, traveled through and systematically tried to learn how to create health and balance in all the areas of your brain. Whether it's for depression, anxiety, irritability, moodiness, addiction, attention, memory, learning, or mysticism, we have looked to every element of our individual mind to try to create health and healing. And then, in this last chapter, we have begun to see how our mind, through its diverse disorders— depression, panic, brain fog, and so on—may actually help let us know intuitively when something is wrong in our own bodies. However, in each and every page of this book, we've mostly only talked about *your* brain, *your* body, *your* mind, and how they affect one another.

True, every once in a while I've alluded to the fact that your emotions, your intuition, or your health may be reactive to people around you. And in the last story in the last chapter, I even talked about how being on a spiritual path, as you try to intertwine your mind with that of the divine, affects your emotional and physical health. Still, when it comes to healing your mind and your body to create wholeness, it's important to realize that the boundaries of your identity as an individual are not distinct. They intertwine with other people in the form of relationships. So you may spend a lot of time working on your emotional and physical health; however, since all of us have some kind of relationship to someone somewhere, their lack of health and happiness ultimately affects our own, whether we like it or not.

Which brings us to the healing aspects of relationships. Relationships to whom? Not just relationships to other people in our family, or a partner, or people at work, or our children, but something outside of ourselves. Perhaps a power greater than ourselves—if you can fathom that? Maybe even something we define as the divine. Whether you're facing depression, panic, moodiness, addiction, a learning disorder, a memory problem, a life-altering health problem, or even cancer, the extreme stress of crisis releases chemicals that alter your brain. The opiates, the cortisol, the norepinephrine, change the properties in the emotional, intuitive, mystical areas in your mind and alter your sense of reality. And perhaps such an event has an adaptive quality in that it rewires your brain for intuition and a capacity to access a higher power—to connect to the divine.

For many, feeling alone is something we try to avoid and have avoided all our lives. For others, having been a black sheep or a pariah, maybe it feels just a little bit safer to be on the fringes of society, so as not to get hurt again. Whether you're a social butterfly or a solitary mystic, all of us at one time or another have the singular experience of loneliness and isolation, the fact that we are alone. And the panic and terror of being thrown into the dark forces us to look for some kind of light. And often that light is the divine. Those moments when we are on a precipice to another world, those moments when we become inextricably separate from others, perhaps facilitate in our mind and body the capacity to become one with spirit. All of us have this machinery within our brains, a built-in intuitive and spiritual connection. And all the aspects of our mind that we've looked at in this book—the brain areas for mood, anxiety, addiction, attention, and memory—we can use in some way in pursuit of mysticism and spirituality.

So at any time during your life when something needs to change and your spirit is speaking to you, you might have just a little whisper of a change in your mind. When your intuition or your spirit is telling you that your life is in danger, you might have just a little bit of change in your body. And in those moments when you are on edge, aggravated, irritable, you might feel that tightening in your gut and that pressure in your chest saying *This isn't enough for my life. I want more.* By achieving emotional clarity with your feeling mind, looking at the facts with your rational mind, and balancing the two in one whole intuitive and spiritual mind, you are capable—all of us are capable—of gaining a mystical and intelligent mind-body perspective, whether it's through prayer and contemplation or physical and emotional grace. And whatever path you choose toward wholeness, you can figure out the steps to heal your mind with medicine, affirmations, and intuition.

The Beginning

APPENDIX A

Energy Centers

CHAKRA/ENERGY CENTER CHART:
CONNECTING THE HEALTH PROBLEM
WITH THE EMOTIONAL SITUATION

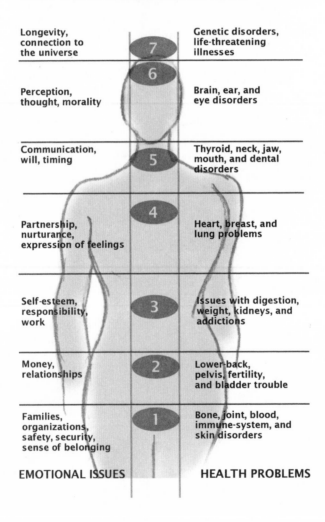

EMOTIONAL ISSUES		HEALTH PROBLEMS
Longevity, connection to the universe	7	Genetic disorders, life-threatening illnesses
	6	
Perception, thought, morality		Brain, ear, and eye disorders
Communication, will, timing	5	Thyroid, neck, jaw, mouth, and dental disorders
	4	
Partnership, nurturance, expression of feelings		Heart, breast, and lung problems
Self-esteem, responsibility, work	3	Issues with digestion, weight, kidneys, and addictions
Money, relationships	2	Lower-back, pelvis, fertility, and bladder trouble
Families, organizations, safety, security, sense of belonging	1	Bone, joint, blood, immune-system, and skin disorders

APPENDIX B

All Is Well Tables

PROBLEM	PROBABLE CAUSE	NEW THOUGHT PATTERN
Abdominal Cramps	Fear. Stopping the process.	I trust the process of life. I am safe.
Abscess	Fermenting thoughts over hurts, slights, and revenge.	I allow my thoughts to be free. The past is over. I'm at peace.
Accidents	Inbility to speak up for the self. Rebellion against authority. Belief in violence.	I release the pattern in me that created this. I am at peace. I am worthwhile.
Aches	Longing for love. Longing to be held.	I love and approve of myself. I am loving and lovable.
Acne	Not accepting the self. Dislike of the self.	I am a Divine expression of life. I love and accept myself where I am right now.
Addictions	Running from the self. Fear. Not knowing how to love the self.	I now discover how wonderful I am. I choose to love and enjoy myself.
Addison's Dis-ease *See: Adrenal Problems*	Severe emotional malnutrition. Anger at the self.	I lovingly take care of my body, my mind, and my emotions.
Adenoids	Family friction, arguments. Child feeling unwelcome, in the way.	This child is wanted and welcomed and deeply loved.
Adrenal Problems *See: Addison's Dis-ease, Cushing's Dis-ease*	Defeatism. No longer caring for the self. Anxiety.	I love and approve of myself. It is safe for me to care for myself.

PROBLEM	PROBABLE CAUSE	NEW THOUGHT PATTERN
Aging Problems	Social beliefs. Old thinking. Fear of being one's self. Rejection of the now.	I love and accept myself at every age. Each moment in life is perfect.
AIDS	Feeling defenseless and hopeless. Nobody cares. A strong belief in not being good enough. Denial of the self. Sexual guilt.	I am part of the universal design. I am important and I am loved by life itself. I am powerful and capable. I love and appreciate all of myself.
Alcoholism	"What's the use?" Feeling of futility, guilt, inadequacy. Self-rejection.	I live in the now. Each moment is new. I choose to see my self-worth. I love and approve of myself.
Allergies *See: Hay Fever*	Who are you allergic to? Denying your own power.	The world is safe and friendly. I am safe. I am at peace with life.
Alzheimer's Dis-ease *See: Dementia, Senility*	Refusal to deal with the world as it is. Hopelessness and helplessness. Anger.	There is always a new and better way for me to experience life. I forgive and release the past. I move into joy.
Amenorrhea *See: Female Problems, Menstrual Problems*	Not wanting to be a woman. Dislike of the self.	I rejoice in who I am. I am a beautiful expression of life, flowing perfectly at all times.
Amnesia	Fear. Running from life. Inability to stand up for the self.	Intelligence, courage, and self-worth are always present. It is safe to be alive.
Amyotrophic Lateral Sclerosis (ALS, or Lou Gehrig's Dis-ease)	Unwillingness to accept self-worth. Denial of success.	I know I am worthwhile. It is safe for me to succeed. Life loves me.
Anemia	"Yes-but" attitude. Lack of joy. Fear of life. Not feeling good enough.	It is safe for me to experience joy in every area of my life. I love life.

PROBLEM	PROBABLE CAUSE	NEW THOUGHT PATTERN
Ankle(s)	Inflexibility and guilt. Ankles represent the ability to receive pleasure.	I deserve to rejoice in life. I accept all the pleasure life has to offer.
Anorectal Bleeding (Hematochezia)	Anger and frustration.	I trust the process of life. Only right and good action is taking place in my life.
Anorexia *See: Appetite, Loss of*	Denying the self. Extreme fear, self-hatred, and rejection.	It is safe to be me. I am wonderful just as I am. I choose to live. I choose joy and self-acceptance.
Anus *See: Hemorrhoids*	Releasing point. Dumping ground.	I easily and comfortably release that which I no longer need.
—Abscess	Anger in relation to what you don't want to release.	It is safe to let go. Only that which I no longer need leaves my body.
—Bleeding *See: Anorectal Bleeding*		
—Fistula	Incomplete releasing of trash. Holding on to the garbage of the past.	It is with love that I totally release the past. I am free. I am love.
—Itching (Pruritus Ani)	Guilt over the past. Remorse.	I lovingly forgive myself. I am free.
—Pain	Guilt. Desire for punishment. Not feeling good enough.	The past is over. I choose to love and approve of myself in the now.
Anxiety	Not trusting the flow and the process of life.	I love and approve of myself and I trust the process of life. I am safe.
Apathy	Resistance to feeling. Deadening of the self. Fear.	It is safe to feel. I open myself to life. I am willing to experience life.
Appendicitis	Fear. Fear of life. Blocking the flow of good.	I am safe. I relax and let life flow joyously.

PROBLEM	PROBABLE CAUSE	NEW THOUGHT PATTERN
Appetite		
—Excessive	Fear. Needing protection. Judging the emotions.	I am safe. It is safe to feel. My feelings are normal and acceptable.
—Loss of *See: Anorexia*	Fear. Protecting the self. Not trusting life.	I love and approve of myself. I am safe. Life is safe and joyous.
Arm(s)	Represents the capacity and ability to hold the experiences of life.	I lovingly hold and embrace my experiences with ease and with joy.
Arteries	Carry the joy of life.	I am filled with joy. It flows through me with every beat of my heart.
Arteriosclerosis	Resistance, tension. Hardened narrow-mindedness. Refusing to see good.	I am completely open to life and to joy. I choose to see with love.
Arthritic Fingers	A desire to punish. Blame. Feeling victimized.	I see with love and understanding. I hold all my experiences up to the light of love.
Arthritis See: Joints	Feeling unloved. Criticism, resentment.	I am love. I now choose to love and approve of myself. I see others with love.
Asphyxiating Attacks *See: Breathing Problems, Hyperventilation*	Fear. Not trusting the process of life. Getting stuck in childhood.	It is safe to grow up. The world is safe. I am safe.
Asthma	*Smother* love. Inability to breathe for one's self. Feeling stifled. Suppressed crying.	It is safe now for me to take charge of my own life. I choose to be free.
—Babies and Children	Fear of life. Not wanting to be here.	This child is safe and loved. This child is welcomed and cherished.
Athlete's Foot	Frustration at not being accepted. Inability to move forward with ease.	I love and approve of myself. I give myself permission to go ahead. It's safe to move.

282

PROBLEM	PROBABLE CAUSE	NEW THOUGHT PATTERN
Attention Deficit Hyperactivity Disorder (ADHD)	Inflexibility. Fear of the world.	Life loves me. I love myself just the way I am. I am free to create a joyous life that works for me. All is well in my world."
Back	Represents the support of life.	I know that life always supports me.
Back Problems		
—Lower	Fear of money. Lack of financial support.	I trust the process of life. All I need is always taken care of. I am safe.
—Middle	Guilt. Stuck in all that stuff back there. "Get off my back."	I release the past. I am free to move forward with love in my heart.
—Upper	Lack of emotional support. Feeling unloved. Holding back love.	I love and approve of myself. Life supports me and loves me.
Bad Breath *See: Halitosis*	Anger and revenge thoughts. Experiences backing up.	I release the past with love. I choose to voice only love.
Balance, Loss of	Scattered thinking. Not centered.	I center myself in safety and accept the perfection of my life. All is well.
Baldness	Fear. Tension. Trying to control everything. Not trusting the process of life.	I am safe. I love and approve of myself. I trust life.
Bed-Wetting (Enuresis)	Fear of parent, usually the father.	This child is seen with love, with compassion, and with understanding. All is well.
Belching	Fear. Gulping life too quickly.	There is time and space for everything I need to do. I am at peace.
Bell's Palsy *See: Palsy, Paralysis*	Extreme control over anger. Unwillingness to express feelings.	It is safe for me to express my feelings. I forgive myself.

PROBLEM	PROBABLE CAUSE	NEW THOUGHT PATTERN
Birth	Represents the entering of this segment of the movie of life.	This baby now begins a joyous and wonderful new life. All is well.
—Defects	Karmic. You selected to come that way. We choose our parents and our children. Unfinished business.	Every experience is perfect for our growth process. I am at peace with where I am.
Bites	Fear. Open to every slight.	I forgive myself and I love myself now and forever more.
—Animal	Anger turned inward. A need for punishment.	I am free.
—Bug	Guilt over small things.	I am free of all irritations. All is well.
Blackheads	Small outbursts of anger.	I calm my thoughts and I am serene.
Bladder Problems (Cystitis)	Anxiety. Holding on to old ideas. Fear of letting go. Being *pissed off*.	I comfortably and easily release the old and welcome the new in my life. I am safe.
Bleeding	Joy running out. Anger. But where?	I am the joy of Life expressing and receiving perfect rhythm.
Bleeding Gums	Lack of joy in the decision made in life.	I trust that right action is always taking place in my life. I am at peace.
Blisters	Resistance. Lack of emotional protection.	I gently flow with life and each new experience. All is well.
Blood	Represents joy in the body, flowing freely.	I am the joy of Life expressing and receiving.
Blood Pressure		
—High (Hypertension)	Long-standing emotional problem not solved.	I joyously release the past. I am at peace.

PROBLEM	PROBABLE CAUSE	NEW THOUGHT PATTERN
—Low	Lack of love as a child. Defeatism. "What's the use? It won't work anyway."	I now choose to live in the ever-joyous NOW. My life is a joy.
Blood Problems *See: Leukemia*	Lack of joy. Lack of circulation of ideas.	Joyous new ideas are circulating freely within me.
—Anemic *See: Anemia*		
—Clotting	Closing down the flow of joy.	I awaken new life within me. I flow.
Body Odor	Fear. Dislike of the self. Fear of others.	I love and approve of myself. I am safe.
Boils (Furuncle) *See: Carbuncle*	Anger. Boiling over. Seething.	I express love and joy and I am at peace.
Bone(s) *See: Skeleton*	Represent the structure of the Universe.	I am well structured and balanced.
Bone Marrow	Represents your deepest beliefs about the self. How you support and care for yourself.	Divine Spirit is in the structure of my life. I am safe, loved, and totally supported.
Bone Problems		
—Breaks/Fractures	Rebelling against authority.	In my world, I am my own authority, for I am the only one who thinks in my mind.
—Deformity *See: Osteomyelitis, Osteoporosis*	Mental pressures and tightness. Muscles can't stretch. Loss of mental mobility.	I breathe in life fully. I relax and trust the flow and the process of life.
Bowels	Represents the release of waste.	Letting go is easy.
—Problems	Fear of letting go of the old and no longer needed.	I freely and easily release the old and joyously welcome the new.
Brain	Represents the computer, the switchboard.	I am the loving operator of my mind.

PROBLEM	PROBABLE CAUSE	NEW THOUGHT PATTERN
—Tumor	Incorrect computerized beliefs. Stubborn. Refusing to change old patterns.	It is easy for me to reprogram the computer of my mind. All of life is change, and my mind is ever new.
Breast(s)	Represents mothering and nurturing and nourishment.	I take in and give out nourishment in perfect balance.
Breast Problems —Cysts, Lumps, Soreness (Mastitis)	A refusal to nourish the self. Putting everyone else first. Overmothering. Overprotection. Overbearing attitudes.	I am important. I count. I now care for and nourish myself with love and with joy. I allow others the freedom to be who they are. We are all safe and free.
Breath	Represents the ability to take in life.	I love life. It is safe to live.
Breathing Problems See: Asphyxiating Attacks, Hyperventilation	Fear or refusal to take in life fully. Not feeling the right to take up space or even exist.	It is my birthright to live fully and freely. I am worth loving. I now choose to live life fully.
Bright's Dis-ease See: Nephritis	Feeling like a kid who can't do it right and is not good enough. A failure. Loss.	I love and approve of myself. I care for me. I am totally adequate at all times.
Bronchitis See: Respiratory Ailments	Inflamed family environment. Arguments and yelling. Sometimes silent.	I declare peace and harmony within me and around me. All is well.
Bruises (Ecchymoses)	The little bumps in life. Self-punishment.	I love and cherish myself. I am kind and gentle with me. All is well.
Bulimia	Hopeless terror. A frantic stuffing and purging of self-hatred.	I am loved and nourished and supported by Life itself. It is safe for me to be alive.

PROBLEM	PROBABLE CAUSE	NEW THOUGHT PATTERN
Bunions	Lack of joy in meeting the experience of life.	I joyously run forward to greet life's wonderful experiences.
Burns	Anger. Burning up. Incensed.	I create only peace and harmony within myself and my environment. I deserve to feel good.
Bursitis	Repressed anger. Wanting to hit someone.	Love relaxes and releases all unlike itself.
Buttocks	Represents power. *Loose buttocks*, loss of power.	I use my power wisely. I am strong. I am safe. All is well.
Calluses	Hardened concepts and ideas. Fear solidified.	It is safe to see and experience new ideas and new ways. I am open and receptive to good.
Cancer	Deep hurt. Long-standing resentment. Deep secret or grief eating away at the self. Carrying hatreds. "What's the use?"	I lovingly forgive and release all of the past. I choose to fill my world with joy. I love and approve of myself.
Candida (Candidiasis) See: *Thrush, Yeast Infections*	Feeling very scattered. Lots of frustration and anger. Demanding and untrusting in relationships. Great takers.	I give myself permission to be all that I can be, and I deserve the very best in life. I love and appreciate myself and others.
Canker Sores	Festering words held back by the lips. Blame.	I create only joyful experiences in my loving world.
Carbuncle See: *Boils*	Poisonous anger about personal injustices.	I release the past and allow time to heal every area of my life.
Carpal-Tunnel Syndrome See: *Wrist*	Anger and frustration at life's seeming injustices.	I now choose to create a life that is joyous and abundant. I am at ease.

PROBLEM	PROBABLE CAUSE	NEW THOUGHT PATTERN
Car Sickness *See: Motion Sickness*	Fear. Bondage. Feeling of being trapped.	I move with ease through time and space. Only love surrounds me.
Cataracts	Inability to see ahead with joy. Dark future.	Life is eternal and filled with joy. I look forward to every moment.
Cellulite	Stored anger and self-punishment.	I forgive others. I forgive myself. I am free to love and enjoy life.
Cerebral Palsy *See: Palsy*	A need to unite the family in an action of love.	I contribute to a united, loving, and peaceful family life. All is well.
Cerebrovascular Accident *See: Stroke*		
Childhood Dis-ease	Belief in calendars and social concepts and false laws. Childish behavior in the adults around them.	This child is Divinely protected and surrounded by love. We claim mental immunity.
Chills	Mental contraction, pulling away and in. Desire to retreat. "Leave me alone."	I am safe and secure at all times. Love surrounds me and protects me. All is well.
Cholelithiasis *See: Gallstones*		
Cholesterol (Atherosclerosis)	Clogging the channels of joy. Fear of accepting joy.	I choose to love life. My channels of joy are wide open. It is safe to receive.
Chronic Dis-eases	A refusal to change. Fear of the future. Not feeling safe.	I am willing to change and to grow. I now create a safe, new future.
Circulation	Represents the ability to feel and express the emotions in positive ways.	I am free to circulate love and joy in every part of my world. I love life.

PROBLEM	PROBABLE CAUSE	NEW THOUGHT PATTERN
Cold Sores (Fever Blisters) *See: Herpes Simplex*	Festering angry words and fear of repressing them.	I only create peaceful experiences because I love myself. All is well.
Colds (Upper-Respiratory Illness) *See: Respiratory Ailments*	Too much going on at once. Mental confusion, disorder. Small hurts. "I get three colds every winter," type of belief.	I allow my mind to relax and be at peace. Clarity and harmony are within me and around me. All is well.
Colic	Mental irritation, impatience, annoyance in the surroundings.	This child responds only to love and having loving thoughts. All is peaceful.
Colon	Fear of letting go. Holding on to the past.	I easily release that which I no longer need. The past is over, and I am free.
Colitis *See: Colon, Intestines, Mucus Colon, Spastic Colitis*	Insecurity. Represents the ease of letting go of that which is over.	I am part of the perfect rhythm and flow of life. All is in Divine right order.
Coma	Fear. Escaping something or someone.	We surround you with safety and love. We create a space for you to heal. You are loved.
Comedones	Small outbursts of anger.	I calm my thoughts and I am serene.
Congestion *See: Bronchitis, Colds, Influenza*		
Conjunctivitis *See: Pinkeye*	Anger and frustration at what you are looking at in life.	I see with the eyes of love. There is a harmonious solution, and I accept it now.
Constipation	Refusing to release old ideas. Stuck in the past. Sometimes stinginess.	As I release the past, the new and fresh and vital enter. I allow life to flow through me.

PROBLEM	PROBABLE CAUSE	NEW THOUGHT PATTERN
Corns	Hardened areas of thought, stubbornly holding on to the pain of the past.	I move forward, free from the past. I am safe, I am free.
Coronary Thrombosis *See: Heart Attack*	Feeling alone and scared. "I'm not good enough. I don't do enough. I'll never make it."	I am one with all of life. The Universe totally supports me. All is well.
Coughs *See: Respiratory Ailments*	A desire to bark at the world. "See me! Listen to me!"	I am noticed and appreciated in the most positive ways. I am loved.
Cramps	Tension. Fear. Gripping, holding on.	I relax and allow my mind to be peaceful.
Croup *See: Bronchitis*		
Crying	Tears are the river of life, shed in joy as well as in sadness and fear.	I am peaceful with all my emotions. I love and approve of myself.
Cushing's Dis-ease *See: Adrenal Problems*	Mental imbalance. Overproduction of crushing ideas. A feeling of being overpowered.	I lovingly balance my mind and my body. I now choose thoughts that make me feel good.
Cuts *See: Injuries, Wounds*	Punishment for not following your own rules.	I create a life filled with rewards.
Cyst(s)	Running the old, painful movie. Nursing hurts. A false growth.	The movies of my mind are beautiful because I choose to make them so. I love me.
Cystic Fibrosis	A thick belief that life won't work for you. "Poor me."	Life loves me, and I love life. I now choose to take in life fully and freely.
Cystitis *See: Bladder Problems*		

PROBLEM	PROBABLE CAUSE	NEW THOUGHT PATTERN
Deafness	Rejection, stubbornness, isolation. What don't you want to hear? "Don't bother me."	I listen to the Divine and rejoice at all that I am able to hear. I am one with all.
Death	Represents leaving the movie of life.	I joyfully move on to new levels of experience. All is well.
Defects	Karmic. You selected to come that way. We choose our parents and our children. Unfinished business.	Every experience is perfect for our growth process. I am at peace with where I am.
Degenerative Disc	Lack of support. Fear of life. Inability to trust.	I am willing to learn to love myself. I allow my love to support me. I am learning to trust life and accept its abundance. It is safe for me to trust.
Dementia *See: Alzheimer's* *Dis-ease, Senility*	A refusal to deal with the world as it is. Hopelessness and anger.	I am in my perfect place, and I am safe at all times.
Depression	Anger you feel you do not have a right to have. Hopelessness.	I now go beyond other people's fears and limitations. I create my life.
Diabetes (Hyperglycemia, Mellitus)	Longing for what might have been. A great need to control. Deep sorrow. No sweetness left.	This moment is filled with joy. I now choose to experience the sweetness of today.
Diarrhea	Fear. Rejection. Running off.	My intake, assimilation, and elimination are in perfect order. I am at peace with life.
Dizziness (Vertigo)	Flighty, scattered thinking. A refusal to look.	I am deeply centered and peaceful in life. It is safe for me to be alive and joyous.

PROBLEM	PROBABLE CAUSE	NEW THOUGHT PATTERN
Dry Eye	Angry eyes. Refusing to see with love. Would rather die than forgive. Being spiteful.	I willingly forgive. I breathe life into my vision and see with compassion and understanding.
Dysentery	Fear and intense anger.	I create peacefulness in my mind, and my body reflects this.
—Amoebic	Believing *they* are out to get you.	I am the power and authority in my world. I am at peace.
—Bacillary	Oppression and hopelessness.	I am filled with life and energy and the joy of living.
Dysmenorrhea *See: Female Problems, Menstrual Problems*	Anger at the self. Hatred of the body or of women.	I love my body. I love myself. I love all my cycles. All is well.
Ear	Represents the capacity to hear.	I hear with love.
Ear Problems	Inability to hear or fully open up your mind to the outside world. Lack of trust.	I now learn to trust my higher self. I release all ideas that are unlike the voice of love.
Earache (Otitis: External/Ear Canal Media/Inner Ear)	Anger. Not wanting to hear. Too much turmoil. Parents arguing.	Harmony surrounds me. I listen with love to the pleasant and the good. I am a center for love.
Ecchymoses *See: Bruises*		
Eczema	Breath-taking antagonism. Mental eruptions.	Harmony and peace, love and joy surround me and indwell me. I am safe and secure.
Edema *See: Holding Fluids, Swelling*	What or who won't you let go of?	I willingly release the past. It is safe for me to let go. I am free now.
Elbow *See: Joints*	Represents changing directions and accepting new experiences.	I easily flow with new experiences, new directions, and new changes.

PROBLEM	PROBABLE CAUSE	NEW THOUGHT PATTERN
Emphysema	Fear of taking in life. Not worthy of living.	It is my birthright to live fully and freely. I love life. I love me.
Endometriosis	Insecurity, disappointment, and frustration. Replacing self-love with sugar. Blamers.	I am both powerful and desirable. It's wonderful to be a woman. I love myself, and I am fulfilled.
Enuresis *See: Bed-Wetting*		
Epilepsy	Sense of persecution. Rejection of life. A feeling of great struggle. Self-violence.	I choose to see life as eternal and joyous. I am eternal and joyous and at peace.
Epstein-Barr Virus	Pushing beyond one's limits. Fear of not being good enough. Draining all inner support. Stress virus.	I relax and recognize my self-worth. I am good enough. Life is easy and joyful.
Exotropia *See: Eye Problems*		
Eye(s)	Represents the capacity to see clearly—past, present, and future.	I see with love and joy.
Eye Problems *See: Sty*	Not liking what you see in your own life.	I now create a life I love to look at.
—Astigmatism	"I" trouble. Fear of really seeing the self.	I am now willing to see my own beauty and magnificence.
—Cataracts	Inability to see ahead with joy. Dark future.	Life is eternal and filled with joy.
—Children	Not wanting to see what is going on in the family.	Harmony and joy and beauty and safety now surround this child.
—Crossed *See: Keratitis*	Not wanting to see what's out there. Crossed purposes.	It is safe for me to see. I am at peace.
—Farsighted (Hyperopia)	Fear of the present.	I am safe in the here and now. I see that clearly.

PROBLEM	PROBABLE CAUSE	NEW THOUGHT PATTERN
—Glaucoma	Stony unforgiveness. Pressure from long-standing hurts. Overwhelmed by it all.	I see with love and tenderness.
—Nearsighted *See: Myopia*	Fear of the future.	I accept Divine guidance and am always safe.
—Wall Eyed (Exotropia)	Fear of looking at the present, right here.	I accept Divine guidance and am always safe.
Face	Represents what we show the world.	It is safe to be me. I express who I am.
Fainting (Vasovagal Attack)	Fear. Can't cope. Blacking out.	I have the power and the strength and knowledge to handle everything in my life.
Fat *See: Overweight*	Oversensitivity. Often represents fear and shows a need for protection. Fear may be a cover for hidden anger and a resistance to forgive.	I am protected by Divine Love. I am always safe and secure. I am willing to grow up and take responsibility for my life. I forgive others and I now create my own life the way I want it. I am safe.
—Arms	Anger at being denied love.	It is safe for me to create all the love I want.
—Belly	Anger at being denied nourishment.	I nourish myself with spiritual food, and I am satisfied and free.
—Hips	Lumps of stubborn anger at the parents.	I am willing to forgive the past. It is safe for me to go beyond my parents' limitations.
—Thighs	Packed childhood anger. Often rage at the father.	I see my father as a loveless child, and I forgive easily. We are both free.
Fatigue	Resistance, boredom. Lack of love for what one does.	I am enthusiastic about life and filled with energy and enthusiasm.

PROBLEM	PROBABLE CAUSE	NEW THOUGHT PATTERN
Feet *See: Foot Problems*	Represents our understanding—of ourselves, of life, of others.	My understanding is clear, and I am willing to change with the times. I am safe.
Female Problems *See: Amenorrhea, Dysmenorrhea, Fibroid Tumors, Leukorrhea, Menstrual Problems, Vaginitis*	Denial of the self. Rejecting femininity. Rejection of the feminine principle.	I rejoice in my femaleness. I love being a woman. I love my body.
Fertility Problems	Fear. Worry about not being good enough. Resistance to the process of life.	I love and cherish my inner child. I love and adore myself. I am the most important person in my life. All is well and I am safe.
Fever	Anger. Burning up.	I am the cool, calm expression of peace and love.
Fever Blisters *See: Cold Sores, Herpes Simplex*		
Fibroid Tumors & Cysts *See: Female Problems*	Nursing a hurt from a partner. A blow to the feminine ego.	I release the pattern in me that attracted this experience. I create only good in my life.
Fingers	Represent the details of life.	I am peaceful with the details of life.
—Thumb	Represents intellect and worry.	My mind is at peace.
—Index Finger	Represents ego and fear.	I am secure.
—Middle Finger	Represents anger and sexuality.	I am comfortable with my sexuality.
—Ring Finger	Represents unions and grief.	I am peacefully loving.
—Little Finger	Represents the family and pretending.	I am myself with the family of Life.
Fistula	Fear. Blockage in the letting-go process.	I am safe. I trust fully in the process of life. Life is for me.

PROBLEM	PROBABLE CAUSE	NEW THOUGHT PATTERN
Flatulence *See: Gas Pains*		
Flu *See: Influenza*		
Food Poisoning	Allowing others to take control. Feeling defenseless.	I have the strength, power, and skill to digest whatever comes my way.
Foot problems	Fear of the future and of not stepping forward in life.	I move forward in life with joy and with ease.
Frigidity	Fear. Denial of pleasure. A belief that sex is bad. Insensitive partners. Fear of father.	It is safe for me to enjoy my own body. I rejoice in being a woman.
Fungus	Stagnating beliefs. Refusing to release the past. Letting the past rule today.	I live in the present moment, joyous and free.
Furuncle *See: Boils*		
Gallstones (Cholelithiasis)	Bitterness. Hard thoughts. Condemning. Pride.	There is joyous release of the past. Life is sweet, and so am I.
Gangrene	Mental morbidity. Drowning of joy with poisonous thoughts.	I now choose harmonious thoughts and let the joy flow freely through me.
Gas Pains (Flatulence)	Gripping. Fear. Undigested ideas.	I relax and let life flow through me with ease.
Gastritis *See: Stomach Problems*	Prolonged uncertainty. A feeling of doom.	I love and approve of myself. I am safe.
Genitals	Represents the masculine and feminine principles.	It is safe to be who I am.
—Problems	Worry about not being good enough.	I rejoice in my own expression of life. I am perfect just as I am. I love and approve of myself.

PROBLEM	PROBABLE CAUSE	NEW THOUGHT PATTERN
Gland(s)	Represent holding stations. Self-starting activity.	I am a creative power in my world.
Glandular Fever *See: Mononucleosis*		
Glandular Problems	Poor distribution of get-up-and-go ideas. Holding yourself back.	I have all the Divine ideas and activity I need. I move forward right now.
Globus Hystericus *See: Lump in Throat*		
Goiter *See: Thyroid*	Hatred for being inflicted upon. Victim. Feeling thwarted in life. Unfulfilled.	I am the power and authority in my life. I am free to be me.
Gonorrhea *See: Venereal Dis-ease*	A need for punishment for being a *bad* person.	I love my body. I love my sexuality. I love me.
Gout	The need to dominate. Impatience, anger.	I am safe and secure. I am at peace with myself and with others.
Gray Hair	Stress. A belief in pressure and strain.	I am at peace and comfortable in every area of my life. I am strong and capable.
Growths	Nursing those old hurts. Building resentments.	I easily forgive. I love myself and will reward myself with thoughts of praise.
Gum Problems	Inability to back up decisions. Wishy-washy about life.	I am a decisive person. I follow through and support myself with love.
Halitosis *See: Bad Breath*	Rotten attitudes, vile gossip, foul thinking.	I speak with gentleness and love. I exhale only the good.

PROBLEM	PROBABLE CAUSE	NEW THOUGHT PATTERN
Hands	Hold and handle. Clutch and grip. Grasping and letting go. Caressing. Pinching. All ways of dealing with experiences.	I choose to handle all my experiences with love and with joy and with ease.
Hay Fever See: Allergies	Emotional congestion. Fear of the calendar. A belief in persecution. Guilt.	I am one with ALL OF LIFE. I am safe at all times.
Headaches See: Migraine Headaches	Invalidating the self. Self-criticism. Fear.	I love and approve of myself. I see myself and what I do with eyes of love. I am safe.
Heart See: Blood	Represents the center of love and security.	My heart beats to the rhythm of love.
—Attack (M.I./ Myocardial Infarction) See: Coronary Thrombosis	Squeezing all the joy out of the heart in favor of money or position, etc.	I bring joy back to the center of my heart. I express love to all.
—Problems	Long-standing emotional problems. Lack of joy. Hardening of the heart. Belief in strain and stress.	Joy. Joy. Joy. I lovingly allow joy to flow through my mind and body and experience.
Heartburn See: Peptic Ulcer, Stomach Problems, Ulcers	Fear. Fear. Fear. Clutching fear.	I breathe freely and fully. I am safe. I trust the process of life.
Hematochezia See: Anorectal Bleeding		
Hemorrhoids See: Anus	Fear of deadlines. Anger of the past. Afraid to let go. Feeling burdened.	I release all that is unlike love. There is time and space for everything I want to do.
Hepatitis See: Liver Problems	Resistance to change. Fear, anger, hatred. Liver is the seat of anger and rage.	My mind is cleansed and free. I leave the past and move forward into the new. All is well.

PROBLEM	PROBABLE CAUSE	NEW THOUGHT PATTERN
Hernia	Ruptured relationships. Strain, burdens, incorrect creative expression.	My mind is gentle and harmonious. I love and approve of myself. I am free to be me.
Herpes (Herpes Genitalis) *See: Venereal Dis-ease*	Mass belief in sexual guilt and the need for punishment. Public shame. Belief in a punishing God. Rejection of the genitals.	My concept of God supports me. I am normal and natural. I rejoice in my own sexuality and in my own body. I am wonderful.
Herpes Simplex (Herpes Labialis) *See: Cold Sores*	Burning to bitch. Bitter words left unspoken.	I think and speak only words of love. I am at peace with life.
Hip(s)	Carries the body in perfect balance. Major thrust in moving forward.	Hip Hip Hooray—there is joy in every day. I am balanced and free.
Hip Problems	Fear of going forward in major decisions. Nothing to move forward to.	I am in perfect balance. I move forward in life with ease and with joy at every age.
Hirsutism	Anger that is covered over. The blanket used is usually fear. A desire to blame. There is often an unwillingness to nurture the self.	I am a loving parent to myself. I am covered with love and approval. It is safe for me to show who I am.
Hives (Urticaria) *See: Rash*	Small, hidden tears. Mountains out of molehills.	I bring peace to every corner of my life.
Hodgkin's Dis-ease	Blame and a tremendous fear of not being good enough. A frantic race to prove one's self until the blood has no substance left to support itself. The joy of life is forgotten in the race for acceptance.	I am perfectly happy to be me. I am good enough just as I am. I love and approve of myself. I am joy expressing and receiving.

PROBLEM	PROBABLE CAUSE	NEW THOUGHT PATTERN
Holding Fluids *See: Edema, Swelling*	What are you afraid of losing?	I willingly release with joy.
Huntington's Dis-ease	Resentment at not being able to change others. Hopelessness.	I release all control to the Universe. I am at peace with myself and with life.
Hyperactivity	Fear. Feeling pressured and frantic.	I am safe. All pressure dissolves. I AM good enough.
Hyperglycemia *See: Diabetes*		
Hyperopia *See: Eye Problems*		
Hypertension *See: Blood Pressure*		
Hyperthyroidism *See: Thyroid*	Rage at being left out.	I am at the center of life, and I approve of myself and all that I see.
Hyperventilation *See: Asphyxiating Attacks, Breathing Problems*	Fear. Resisting change. Not trusting the process.	I am safe everywhere in the Universe. I love myself and trust the process of life.
Hypoglycemia	Overwhelmed by the burdens in life. "What's the use?"	I now choose to make my life light and easy and joyful.
Hypothyroidism *See: Thyroid*	Giving up. Feeling hopelessly stifled.	I create a new life with new rules that totally support me.
Ileitis (Crohn's Dis-ease, Regional Enteritis)	Fear. Worry. Not feeling good enough.	I love and approve of myself. I am doing the best I can. I am wonderful. I am at peace.
Impotence	Sexual pressure, tension, guilt. Social beliefs. Spite against a previous mate. Fear of mother.	I now allow the full power of my sexual principle to operate with ease and with joy.

PROBLEM	PROBABLE CAUSE	NEW THOUGHT PATTERN
Incontinence	Emotional overflow. Years of controlling the emotions.	I am willing to feel. It is safe for me to express my emotions. I love myself.
Incurable	Cannot be cured by outer means at this point. We must go within to effect the cure. It came from nowhere and will go back to nowhere.	Miracles happen every day. I go within to dissolve the pattern that created this, and I now accept a Divine healing. And so it is!
Indigestion	Gut-level fear, dread, anxiety. Griping and grunting.	I digest and assimilate all new experiences peacefully and joyously.
Infection *See: Viral Infection*	Irritation, anger, annoyance.	I choose to be peaceful and harmonious.
Infertility *See: Fertility Problems*		
Inflammation *See: "Itis"*	Fear. Seeing red. Inflamed thinking.	My thinking is peaceful, calm, and centered.
Influenza *See: Respiratory Ailments*	Response to mass negativity and beliefs. Fear. Belief in statistics.	I am beyond group beliefs or the calendar. I am free from all congestion and influence.
Ingrown Toenail	Worry and guilt about your right to move forward.	It is my Divine right to take my own direction in life. I am safe. I am free.
Injuries *See: Cuts, Wounds*	Anger at the self. Feeling guilty.	I now release anger in positive ways. I love and appreciate myself.
Insanity (Psychiatric Illness)	Fleeing from the family. Escapism, withdrawal. Violent separation from life.	This mind knows its true identity and its creative point of Divine Self-Expression.
Insomnia	Fear. Not trusting the process of life. Guilt.	I lovingly release the day and slip into peaceful sleep, knowing tomorrow will take care of itself.

PROBLEM	PROBABLE CAUSE	NEW THOUGHT PATTERN
Intestines *See: Colon*	Assimilation. Absorption. Elimination with ease.	I easily assimilate and absorb all that I need to know and release the past with joy.
Itching (Pruritis)	Desires that go against the grain. Unsatisfied. Remorse. Itching to get out or get away.	I am at peace just where I am. I accept my good, knowing that all my needs and desires will be fulfilled.
"Itis" *See: Inflammation*	Anger and frustration about conditions you are looking at in your life.	I am willing to change all patterns of criticism. I love and approve of myself.
Jaundice *See: Liver Problems*	Internal and external prejudice. Unbalanced reason.	I feel tolerance and compassion and love for all people, myself included.
Jaw Problems (Temporomandibular Joint/TMJ Syndrome)	Anger. Resentment. Desire for revenge.	I am willing to change the patterns in me that created this condition. I love and approve of myself. I am safe.
Joints *See: Arthritis, Elbow, Knee, Shoulders*	Represent changes in direction in life and the ease of these movements.	I easily flow with change. My life is Divinely guided, and I am always going in the best direction.
Keratitis *See: Eye Problems*	Extreme anger. A desire to hit those or what you see.	I allow the love from my own heart to heal all that I see. I choose peace. All is well in my world.
Kidney Problems	Criticism, disappointment, failure. Shame. Reacting like a little kid.	Divine right action is always taking place in my life. Only good comes from each experience. It is safe to grow up.
Kidney Stones	Lumps of undissolved anger.	I dissolve all past problems with ease.
Knee *See: Joints*	Represents pride and ego.	I am flexible and flowing.

PROBLEM	PROBABLE CAUSE	NEW THOUGHT PATTERN
Knee Problems	Stubborn ego and pride. Inability to bend. Fear. Inflexibility. Won't give in.	Forgiveness. Understanding. Compassion. I bend and flow with ease, and all is well.
Laryngitis	So mad you can't speak. Fear of speaking up. Resentment of authority.	I am free to ask for what I want. It is safe to express myself. I am at peace.
Left Side of Body	Represents receptivity, taking in, feminine energy, women, the mother.	My feminine energy is beautifully balanced.
Leg(s)	Carry us forward in life.	Life is for me.
Leg Problems —Lower	Fear of the future. Not wanting to move.	I move forward with confidence and joy, knowing that all is well in my future.
Leprosy	Inability to handle life at all. A long-held belief in not being good enough or clean enough.	I rise above all limitations. I am Divinely guided and inspired. Love heals all life.
Leukemia *See: Blood Problems*	Brutally killing inspiration. "What's the use?"	I move beyond past limitations into the freedom of the now. It is safe to be me.
Leukorrhea *See: Female Problems, Vaginitis*	A belief that women are powerless over the opposite sex. Anger at a mate.	I create all my experiences. I am the power. I rejoice in my femaleness. I am free.
Liver	Seat of anger and primitive emotions.	Love and peace and joy are what I know.
Liver Problems *See: Hepatitis, Jaundice*	Chronic complaining. Justifying fault-finding to deceive yourself. Feeling bad.	I choose to live through the open space in my heart. I look for love and find it everywhere.
Lockjaw *See: Tetanus*	Anger. A desire to control. A refusal to express feelings.	I trust the process of my life. I easily ask for what I want. Life supports me.

PROBLEM	PROBABLE CAUSE	NEW THOUGHT PATTERN
Lou Gehrig's Dis-ease *See: Amyotrophic Lateral Sclerosis*		
Lump in Throat (Globus Hystericus)	Fear. Not trusting the process of life.	I am safe. I trust that Life is here for me. I express myself freely and joyously.
Lung	The ability to take in life.	I take in life in perfect balance.
—Problems *See: Pneumonia*	Depression. Grief. Fear of taking in life. Not feeling worthy of living life fully.	I have the capacity to take in the fullness of life. I lovingly live life to the fullest.
Lupus (Erythematosus)	A giving up. Better to die than stand up for one's self. Anger and punishment.	I speak up for myself freely and easily. I claim my own power. I love and approve of myself. I am free and safe.
Lymph Problems	A warning that the mind needs to be recentered on the essentials of life. Love and joy.	I am now totally centered in the love and joy of being alive. I flow with life. Peace of mind is mine.
Malaria	Out of balance with nature and with life.	I am united and balanced with all of my life. I am safe.
Mastitis *See: Breast Problems*		
Mastoiditis	Anger and frustration. A desire not to hear what is going on. Usually in children. Fear infecting the understanding.	Divine peace and harmony surround and indwell me. I am an oasis of peace and love and joy. All is well in my world.
Mellitus *See: Diabetes*		
Menopause Problems	Fear of no longer being wanted. Fear of aging. Self-rejection. Not feeling good enough.	I am balanced and peaceful in all changes of cycles, and I bless my body with love.

PROBLEM	PROBABLE CAUSE	NEW THOUGHT PATTERN
Menstrual Problems *See: Amenorrhea, Dysmenorrhea, Female Problems*	Rejection of one's femininity. Guilt, fear. Belief that the genitals are sinful or dirty.	I accept my full power as a woman and accept all my bodily processes as normal and natural. I love and approve of myself.
Migraine Headaches *See: Headaches*	Dislike of being driven. Resisting the flow of life. Sexual fears. (Can usually be relieved by masturbation.)	I relax into the flow of life and let life provide all that I need easily and comfortably. Life is for me.
Miscarriage (Abortion, Spontaneous)	Fear. Fear of the future. "Not now—later." Inappropriate timing.	Divine right action is always taking place in my life. I love and approve of myself. All is well.
Mono, Mononucleosis (Pfeiffer's Dis-ease, Glandular Fever)	Anger at not receiving love and appreciation. No longer caring about the self.	I love and appreciate and take care of myself. I am enough.
Motion Sickness *See: Car Sickness, Seasickness*	Fear. Fear of not being in control.	I am always in control of my thoughts. I am safe. I love and approve of myself.
Mouth	Represents taking in of new ideas and nourishment.	I nourish myself with love.
—Problems	Set opinions. Closed mind. Incapacity to take in new ideas.	I welcome new ideas and new concepts and prepare them for digestion and assimilation.
Mucus Colon *See: Colitis, Colon, Intestines, Spastic Colitis*	Layered deposits of old, confused thoughts clogging the channel of elimination. Wallowing in the gummed mire of the past.	I release and dissolve the past. I am a clear thinker. I live now in peace and joy.
Multiple Sclerosis	Mental hardness, hard-heartedness, iron will, inflexibility. Fear.	By choosing loving, joyous thoughts, I create a loving, joyous world. I am safe and free.

PROBLEM	PROBABLE CAUSE	NEW THOUGHT PATTERN
Muscles	Resistance to new experiences. Muscles represent our ability to move in life.	I experience life as a joyous dance.
Muscular Dystrophy	"It's not worth growing up."	I go beyond my parents' limitations. I am free to be the best me I can.
Myocardial Infarction *See: Heart Attack*		
Myopia *See: Eye Problems*	Fear of the future. Not trusting what is ahead.	I accept Divine guidance and am always safe.
Nail(s)	Represents protection.	I reach out safely.
Nail Biting	Frustration. Eating away at the self. Spite of a parent.	It is safe for me to grow up. I now handle my own life with joy and with ease.
Narcolepsy	Can't cope. Extreme fear. Wanting to get away from it all. Not wanting to be here.	I rely on Divine wisdom and guidance to protect me at all times. I am safe.
Nausea	Fear. Rejecting an idea or experience.	I am safe. I trust the process of life to bring only good to me.
Nearsightedness *See: Eye Problems, Myopia*		
Neck (Cervical Spine)	Represents flexibility. The ability to see what's back there.	I am peaceful with life.
Neck Problems	Refusing to see other sides of a question. Stubbornness, inflexibility.	It is with flexibility and ease that I see all sides of an issue. There are endless ways of doing things and seeing things. I am safe.
Nephritis *See: Bright's Disease*	Overreaction to disappointment and failure.	Only right action is taking place in my life. I release the old and welcome the new. All is well.

PROBLEM	PROBABLE CAUSE	NEW THOUGHT PATTERN
Nerves	Represent communication. Receptive reporters.	I communicate with ease and with joy.
Nervous Breakdown	Self-centeredness. Jamming the channels of communication.	I open my heart and create only loving communication. I am safe. I am well.
Nervousness	Fear, anxiety, struggle, rushing. Not trusting the process of life.	I am on an endless journey through eternity, and there is plenty of time. I communicate with my heart. All is well.
Neuralgia	Punishment for guilt. Anguish over communication.	I forgive myself. I love and approve of myself. I communicate with love.
Nodules	Resentment and frustration and hurt ego over career.	I release the pattern of delay within me, and I now allow success to be mine.
Nose	Represents self-recognition.	I recognize my own intuitive ability.
—Bleeds	A need for recognition. Feeling unrecognized and unnoticed. Crying for love.	I love and approve of myself. I recognize my own true worth. I am wonderful.
—Runny	Asking for help. Inner crying.	I love comfort in ways that are pleasing to me.
—Stuffy	Not recognizing the self-worth.	I love and appreciate myself.
Numbness (Paresthesia)	Withholding love and consideration. Going dead mentally.	I share my feelings and my love. I respond to love in everyone.
Osteomyelitis *See: Bone Problems*	Anger and frustration at the very structure of life. Feeling unsupported.	I am peaceful with and trust the process of life. I am safe and secure.
Osteoporosis *See: Bone Problems*	Feeling there is no support left in life.	I stand up for myself, and Life supports me in unexpected, loving ways.

PROBLEM	PROBABLE CAUSE	NEW THOUGHT PATTERN
Ovaries	Represent point of creation. Creativity.	I am balanced in my creative flow.
Overweight *See: Fat*	Fear, need for protection. Running away from feelings. Insecurity, self-rejection. Seeking fulfillment.	I am at peace with my own feelings. I am safe where I am. I create my own security. I love and approve of myself.
Paget's Dis-ease	Feeling there is no longer any foundation to build on. "Nobody cares."	I know I am supported by Life in grand and glorious ways. Life loves me and cares for me.
Pain	Guilt. Guilt always seeks punishment.	I lovingly release the past. They are free and I am free. All is well in my heart now.
Palsy *See: Bell's Palsy, Cerebral Palsy, Parkinson's Dis-ease*	Paralyzing thoughts. Getting stuck.	I am a free thinker, and I have wonderful experiences with ease and with joy.
Pancreas	Represents the sweetness of life.	My life is sweet.
Pancreatitis	Rejection. Anger and frustration because life seems to have lost its sweetness.	I love and approve of myself, and I alone create sweetness and joy in my life.
Panic	Fear. Inability to move with the flow of life.	I am capable and strong. I can handle all situations in my life. I know what to do.
Paralysis *See: Palsy*	Fear. Terror. Escaping a situation or person. Resistance.	I am one with all of life. I am totally adequate for all situations.
Parasites	Giving power to others, letting them take over.	I lovingly take back my power and eliminate all interference.
Parkinson's Dis-ease *See: Palsy*	Fear and an intense desire to control everything and everyone.	I relax knowing I am safe. Life trusts me, and I trust the process of life.

PROBLEM	PROBABLE CAUSE	NEW THOUGHT PATTERN
Peptic Ulcer *See: Heartburn, Stomach Problems, Ulcers*	Fear. A belief that you are not good enough. Anxious to please.	I love and approve of myself. I am at peace with myself. I am wonderful.
Periodontitis *See: Pyorrhea*		
Petit Mal *See: Epilepsy*		
Pfeiffer's Dis-ease *See: Mononucleosis*		
Phlebitis	Anger and frustration. Blaming others for the limitations and lack of joy in life.	Joy now flows freely within me, and I am at peace with life.
Piles *See: Hemorrhoids*		
Pimples *See: Blackheads, Whiteheads*	Small outbursts of anger.	I calm my thoughts, and I am serene.
Pinkeye *See: Conjunctivitis*	Anger and frustration. Not wanting to see.	I release the need to be right. I am at peace. I love and approve of myself.
Pituitary Gland	Represents the control center.	My mind and body are in perfect balance. I control my thoughts.
Plantar Wart	Anger at the very basis of your understanding. Spreading frustration about the future.	I move forward with confidence and ease. I trust and flow with the process of life.
Pneumonia *See: Lung Problems*	Desperate. Tired of life. Emotional wounds that are not allowed to heal.	I freely take in Divine ideas that are filled with the breath and intelligence of Life. This is a new moment.
Poison Ivy	Feeling defenseless and open to attack.	I am powerful, safe, and secure. All is well.
Poison Oak *See: Poison Ivy*		

PROBLEM	PROBABLE CAUSE	NEW THOUGHT PATTERN
Polio	Paralyzing jealously. A desire to stop someone.	There is enough for everyone. I create my good and my freedom with loving thoughts.
Post-Nasal Drip	Inner crying. Childish tears. Victim.	I acknowledge and accept that I am the creative power in my world. I now choose to enjoy my life.
Premenstrual Syndrome (PMS)	Allowing confusion to reign. Giving power to outside influences. Rejection of the feminine processes.	I now take charge of my mind and my life. I am a powerful, dynamic woman! Every part of my body functions perfectly. I love me.
Prostate	Represents the masculine principle.	I accept and rejoice in my masculinity.
Prostate Problems	Mental fears weaken the masculinity. Giving up. Sexual pressure and guilt. Belief in aging.	I love and approve of myself. I accept my own power. I am forever young in spirit.
Pruritus *See: Itching*		
Pruritus Ani *See: Anus*		
Psoriasis *See: Skin Problems*	Fear of being hurt. Deadening the senses of the self. Refusing to accept responsibility for your own feelings.	I am alive to the joys of living. I deserve and accept the very best in life. I love and approve of myself.
Psychiatric Illness *See: Insanity*		
Pubic Bone	Represents genital protection.	My sexuality is safe.
Pyelonephritis See: Urinary Infections		
Pyorrhea (Periodontitis)	Anger at the inability to make decisions. Wishy-washy people.	I approve of myself, and my decisions are always perfect for me.

PROBLEM	PROBABLE CAUSE	NEW THOUGHT PATTERN
Quinsy (Peritonsillar Abscess) *See: Sore Throat, Tonsillitis*	A strong belief that you cannot speak up for yourself and ask for your needs.	It is my birthright to have my needs met. I now ask for what I want with love and with ease.
Rabies	Anger. A belief that violence is the answer.	I am surrounded and indwelled with peace.
Rash *See: Hives*	Irritation over delays. Babyish way to get attention.	I love and approve of myself. I am at peace with the process of life.
Rectum *See: Anus*		
Respiratory Ailments *See: Bronchitis, Colds, Coughs, Influenza*	Fear of taking in life fully.	I am safe. I love my life.
Rheumatism	Feeling victimized. Lack of love. Chronic bitterness. Resentment.	I create my own experiences. As I love and approve of myself and others, my experiences get better and better.
Rheumatoid Arthritis	Deep criticism of authority. Feeling very put upon.	I am my own authority. I love and approve of myself. Life is good.
Rickets	Emotional malnutrition. Lack of love and security.	I am secure and am nourished by the love of the Universe itself.
Right Side of Body	Giving out, letting go, masculine energy, men, the father.	I balance my masculine energy easily and effortlessly.
Ringworm	Allowing others to get under your skin. Not feeling good enough or clean enough.	I love and approve of myself. No person, place, or thing has any power over me. I am free.
Root Canal *See: Teeth*	Can't bite into anything anymore. Root beliefs being destroyed.	I create firm foundations for myself and for my life. I choose my beliefs to support me joyously.

PROBLEM	PROBABLE CAUSE	NEW THOUGHT PATTERN
Round Shoulders *See: Shoulders, Spinal Curvature*	Carrying the burdens of life. Helpless and hopeless.	I stand tall and free. I love and approve of me. My life gets better every day.
Sagging Lines	Sagging lines on the face come from sagging thoughts in the mind. Resentment of life.	I express the joy of living and allow myself to enjoy every moment of every day totally. I become young again.
Scabies	Infected thinking. Allowing others to get under your skin.	I am the living, loving, joyous expression of life. I am my own person.
Sciatica	Being hypocritical. Fear of money and of the future.	I move into my greater good. My good is everywhere, and I am secure and safe.
Scleroderma	Protecting the self from life. Not trusting yourself to be there and to take care of yourself.	I relax completely for I now know I am safe. I trust life and I trust myself.
Scoliosis *See: Round Shoulders, Spinal Curvature*		
Scratches	Feeling life tears at you, life is a rip-off, and that you are being ripped off.	I am grateful for life's generosity to me. I am blessed.
Seasickness *See: Motion Sickness*	Fear. Fear of death. Lack of control.	I am totally safe in the Universe. I am at peace everywhere. I trust Life.
Seizures	Running away from the family, from the self, or from life.	I am at home in the Universe. I am safe and secure and understood.

PROBLEM	PROBABLE CAUSE	NEW THOUGHT PATTERN
Senility *See: Alzheimer's Dis-ease*	Returning to the so-called safety of childhood. Demanding care and attention. A form of control of those around you. Escapism.	Divine protection. Safety. Peace. The intelligence of the Universe operates on every level of life.
Shin(s)	Breaking down ideals. Shins represent the standards of life.	I live up to my highest standards with love and with joy.
Shingles (Varicella)	Waiting for the other shoe to drop. Fear and tension. Too sensitive.	I am relaxed and peaceful because I trust in the process of life. All is well in my world.
Shoulders *See: Joints, Round Shoulders*	Represent our ability to carry out experiences in life joyously. We make life a burden by our attitude.	I choose to allow all my experiences to be joyous and loving.
Sickle-Cell Anemia	A belief that one is not good enough, which destroys the very joy of life.	This child lives and breathes in the joy of life and is nourished by love. God works miracles every day.
Sinus Problems (Sinusitis)	Irritation to one person, someone close.	I declare peace and harmony indwell me and surround me at all times. All is well
Skeleton *See: Bones*	Crumbling of structure. Bones represent the structure of your life.	I am strong and sound. I am well structured.
Skin	Protects our individuality. A sense organ.	I feel safe to be me.
Skin Problems *See: Hives, Psoriasis, Rash*	Anxiety, fear. Old, buried guck. I am being threatened.	I lovingly protect myself with thoughts of joy and peace. The past is forgiven and forgotten. I am free in this moment.

PROBLEM	PROBABLE CAUSE	NEW THOUGHT PATTERN
Slipped Disc	Feeling totally unsupported by life. Indecisive.	Life supports all of my thoughts; therefore, I love and approve of myself and all is well.
Snoring	Stubborn refusal to let go of old patterns.	I release all that is unlike love and joy in my mind. I move from the past into the new and fresh and vital.
Solar Plexus	Gut reactions. Center of our intuitive power.	I trust my inner voice. I am strong, wise, and powerful.
Sores	Unexpressed anger that settles in.	I express my emotions in joyous, positive ways.
Sore Throat See: Quinsy, Throat, Tonsillitis	Holding in angry words. Feeling unable to express the self.	I release all restrictions, and I am free to be me.
Spasms	Tightening our thoughts through fear.	I release, I relax, and I let go. I am safe in life.
Spastic Colitis See: Colitis, Colon, Intestines, Mucus Colon	Fear of letting go. Insecurity.	It is safe for me to live. Life will always provide for me. All is well.
Spinal Curvature (Scoliosis Kyphosis) See: Round Shoulders	The inability to flow with the support of Life. Fear and trying to hold on to old ideas. Not trusting life. Lack of integrity. No courage of conviction.	I release all fears. I now trust the process of life. I know that life is for me. I stand straight and tall with love.
Spinal Meningitis	Inflamed thinking and rage at life.	I release all blame and accept the peacefulness and joy of life.
Spine	Flexible support of life.	I am supported by Life.
Spleen	Obsessions. Being obsessed about things.	I love and approve of myself. I trust the process of life to be there for me. I am safe. All is well.

PROBLEM	PROBABLE CAUSE	NEW THOUGHT PATTERN
Sprains	Anger and resistance. Not wanting to move in a certain direction in life.	I trust the process of life to take me to only my highest good. I am at peace.
Sterility	Fearful and resistant to the process of life, OR not needing to go through the parenting experience.	I trust in the process of life. I am always in the right place, doing the right thing, at the right time. I love and approve of myself.
Stiff Neck *See: Neck Problems*	Unbending bullheadedness.	It is safe to see other viewpoints.
Stiffness	Rigid, stiff thinking.	I am safe enough to be flexible in my mind.
Stomach	Holds nourishment. Digests ideas.	I digest life with ease.
Stomach Problems *See: Gastritis, Heartburn, Peptic Ulcer, Ulcers*	Dread. Fear of the new. Inability to assimilate the new.	Life agrees with me. I assimilate the new every moment of every day. All is well.
Stroke (Cerebrovascular Accident/CVA)	Giving up. Resistance. "Rather die than change." Rejection of life.	Life is change, and I adapt easily to the new. I accept life—past, present, and future.
Stuttering	Insecurity. Lack of self-expression. Not being allowed to cry.	I am free to speak up for myself. I am now secure in my own expression. I communicate only with love.
Sty *See: Eye Problems*	Looking at life through angry eyes. Angry at someone.	I choose to see everyone and everything with joy and love.
Suicide	See life only in black and white. Refusal to see another way out.	I live in the totality of possibilities. There is always another way. I am safe.
Swelling *See: Edema, Holding Fluids*	Being stuck in thinking. Clogged, painful ideas.	My thoughts flow freely and easily. I move through ideas with ease.

PROBLEM	PROBABLE CAUSE	NEW THOUGHT PATTERN
Syphilis *See: Venereal Dis-ease*	Giving away your power and effectiveness.	I decide to be me. I approve of myself as I am.
Tapeworm	Strong belief in being a victim or unclean. Helpless to the seeming attitudes of others.	Others only reflect the good feelings I have about myself. I love and approve of all that I am.
Teeth	Represent decisions.	
—Decay	Inability to make decisions. Tendency to give up easily.	I fill my decisions with love and compassion. My new decisions support me and strengthen me. I have new ideas and put them into action. I am safe in my new decisions.
—Problems	Long-standing indecisiveness. Inability to break down ideas for analysis and decisions.	I make decisions based on the principles of truth, and I rest securely knowing that only right action is taking place in my life.
Temporomandibular Joint *See: Jaw Problems*		
Testicles	Masculine principles. Masculinity.	It is safe to be a man.
Tetanus *See: Lockjaw*	A need to release angry, festering thoughts.	I allow the love from my own heart to wash through me and cleanse and heal every part of my body and my emotions.
Throat	Avenue of expression. Channel of creativity.	I open my heart and sing the joys of love.

PROBLEM	PROBABLE CAUSE	NEW THOUGHT PATTERN
—Problems *See: Sore Throat*	The inability to speak up for one's self. Swallowed anger. Stifled creativity. Refusal to change.	It's okay to make noise. I express myself freely and joyously. I speak up for myself with ease. I express my creativity. I am willing to change.
Thrush *See: Candida, Mouth, Yeast Infections*	Anger over making the *wrong* decisions.	I lovingly accept my decisions, knowing I am free to change. I am safe.
Thymus	Master gland of the immune system. Feeling attacked by Life. *They* are out to get me.	My loving thoughts keep my immune system strong. I am safe inside and out. I hear myself with love.
Thyroid *See: Goiter, Hyperthyroidism, Hypothyroidism*	Humiliation. "I never get to do what I want to do. When is it going to be my turn?"	I move beyond old limitations and now allow myself to express freely and creatively.
Tics, Twitches	Fear. A feeling of being watched by others.	I am approved of by all Life. All is well. I am safe.
Tinnitus	Refusal to listen. Not hearing the inner voice. Stubbornness.	I trust my Higher Self. I listen with love to my inner voice. I release all that is unlike the action of love.
Toes	Represent the minor details of the future.	All details take care of themselves.
Tongue	Represents the ability to taste the pleasures of life with joy.	I rejoice in all of my life's bountiful givingness.
Tonsillitis *See: Quinsy, Sore Throat*	Fear. Repressed emotions. Stifled creativity.	My good now flows freely. Divine ideas express through me. I am at peace.

PROBLEM	PROBABLE CAUSE	NEW THOUGHT PATTERN
Tooth Problems *See: Root Canal*	Long-standing indecisiveness. Inability to break down ideas for analysis and decisions.	I make my decisions based on the principles of truth, and I rest securely, knowing that only right action is taking place in my life.
Tuberculosis	Wasting away from selfishness. Possessive. Cruel thoughts. Revenge.	As I love and approve of myself, I create a joyful, peaceful world to live in.
Tumors	Nursing old hurts and shocks. Building remorse.	I lovingly release the past and turn my attention to this new day. All is well.
Ulcers *See: Heartburn, Peptic Ulcer, Stomach Problems*	Fear. A strong belief that you are not good enough. What is eating away at you?	I love and approve of myself. I am at peace. I am calm. All is well.
Urethritis	Angry, emotions. Being pissed off. Blame.	I only create joyful experiences in my life.
Urinary infections (Cystitis, Pyelonephritis)	Pissed off. Usually at the opposite sex or a lover. Blaming others.	I release the pattern in my consciousness that created this condition. I am willing to change. I love and approve of myself.
Urticaria *See: Hives*		
Uterus	Represents the home of creativity.	I am at home in my body.
Vaginitis *See: Female Problems, Leukorrhea*	Anger at a mate. Sexual guilt. Punishing the self.	Others mirror the love and self-approval I have for myself. I rejoice in my sexuality.
Varicella *See: Shingles*		

PROBLEM	PROBABLE CAUSE	NEW THOUGHT PATTERN
Varicose Veins	Standing in a situation you hate. Discouragement. Feeling overworked and overburdened.	I stand in truth and live and move in joy. I love Life, and circulate freely.
Vasovagal Attack *See: Fainting*		
Venereal Dis-ease *See: AIDS, Gonorrhea, Herpes, Syphilis*	Sexual guilt. Need for punishment. Believe that the genitals are sinful or dirty. Abusing another.	I lovingly and joyously accept my sexuality and its expression. I accept only thoughts that support me and make me feel good.
Vertigo *See: Dizziness*		
Viral Infections *See: Infection*	Lack of joy flowing through life. Bitterness.	I lovingly allow joy to flow freely in my life. I love me.
Vitiligo	Feeling completely outside of things. Not belonging. Not one of the group.	I am at the very center of Life, and I am totally connected in Love.
Vomiting	Violent rejection of ideas. Fear of the new.	I digest life safely and joyously. Only good comes to me and through me.
Vulva	Represents vulnerability.	It is safe to be vulnerable.
Warts	Little expressions of hate. Belief in ugliness.	I am the love and the beauty of Life in full expression.
Weakness	A need for mental rest.	I give my mind a joyous vacation.
Whiteheads *See: Pimples*	Hiding ugliness.	I accept myself as beautiful and loved.
Wisdom Tooth, Impacted	Not giving yourself mental space to create a firm foundation.	I open my consciousness to the expansion of life. There is plenty of space for me to grow and to change.

PROBLEM	PROBABLE CAUSE	NEW THOUGHT PATTERN
Wounds *See: Cuts, Injuries*	Anger and guilt at the self.	I forgive myself, and I choose to love myself.
Wrist	Represents movement and ease.	I handle all my experiences with wisdom, with love, and with ease.
Yeast Infections *See: Candida, Thrush*	Denying your own needs. Not supporting yourself.	I now choose to support myself in loving, joyous ways.

ENDNOTES

Chapter 1: Depression

1. Marsha M. Linehan, *Skills Training Manual for Treating Borderline Personality Disorder*, 1st ed. (New York: Guilford Press, 1993), 145–147; and Mona Lisa Schulz, *The New Feminine Brain* (New York: Free Press, 2005), 139–140.

2. Jaak Panksepp, *Affective Neuroscience: The Foundations of Human and Animal Emotions* (New York: Oxford University Press, 1998), 192–196; and Richard Bandler, "Brain mechanisms of aggression as revealed by electrical and chemical stimulation: suggestion of a central role for the midbrain periaqueductal grey region," in *Progress in Psychobiology and Physiological Psychology*, vol. 13, ed. Alan N. Epstein and Adrian R. Morrison (San Diego: Academic Press, 1998), 67–154.

3. Michael St. Clair, *Object Relations and Self Psychology: An Introduction* (Monterey, CA: Brooks/Cole, 1986), 98.

4. Katty Kay and Claire Shipman, *The Confidence Code: The Science and Art of Self-Assurance—What Women Should Know* (New York: HarperCollins, 2014).

5. Petra Hoen et al., "Depression and cardiovascular disease progression: epidemiology, mechanisms, and treatment," in *Stress and Cardiovascular Disease*, ed. Paul Hjemdahl et al. (London: Springer-Verlag, 2012), 211–233; N. Müller et al., "The cyclooxygenase-2 inhibitor celecoxib has therapeutic effects in major depressions: results of a double-blind, randomized, placebo controlled, add-on pilot study to reboxetine," *Molecular Psychiatry* 11, no. 7 (2006), 680–684; J. Mendlewicz et al., "Shortened onset of action of antidepressants in major depression using acetylsalicylic acid augmentation: a pilot open-label study," *International Clinical Psychopharmacology* 21, no. 4 (2006), 227–231; and N. Brunello et al., "Acetylsalicylic acid accelerates the antidepressant effects of fluoxetine in the chronic escape deficit model of depression," *International Clinical Psychopharmacology* 21, no. 4 (2006), 219–225.

6. G. I. Papakostas et al., "L-methylfolate as adjunctive therapy for SSRI-resistant major depression: results of two randomized, double-blind, parallel-sequential

trials," *American Journal of Psychiatry* 169, no. 12 (December 2012), 1267–1274.

7. B. Kim et al., "Follicle-stimulating hormone (FSH), current suicidal ideation and attempt in female patients with major depressive disorder," *Psychiatry Research* 210, no. 3 (December 2013), 951–956.

CHAPTER 2: ANXIETY

1. G. M. Slavich et al., "Neural sensitivity to social rejection is associated with inflammatory responses to social stress," *Proceedings of the National Academy of Sciences of the United States of America* 107, no. 33 (August 17, 2010), 14817–14822; and Bessel A. van der Kolk et al., eds., *Traumatic Stress: The Effects of Overwhelming Experience on Mind, Body, and Society* (New York: Guilford Press, 2006).

2. B. Labonté et al., "Genome-wide epigenetic regulation by early-life trauma," *Archives of General Psychiatry* 69, no. 7 (July 2012), 722–731.

3. J. D. Bremner, "Brain imaging in anxiety disorders," *Expert Review of Neurotherapeutics* 4, no. 2 (March 2004), 275–284.

4. Linehan, *Skills Training Manual for Treating Borderline Personality Disorder*.

5. J. A. Coan et al., "Lending a hand: social regulation of the neural response to threat," *Psychological Science* 17, no. 12 (December 2006), 1032–1039.

CHAPTER 3: ADDICTION

1. C. P. O'Brien et al., "Conditioned narcotic withdrawal in humans," *Science* 195 (March 11, 1977), 1000–1002; S. Siegel et al., "Heroin 'overdose' death: contribution of drug-associated environmental cues," *Science* 216 (1982), 436–437; P. W. Kalivas and N. D. Volkow, "The neural basis of addiction: a pathology of motivation and choice," *American Journal of Psychiatry* 162 (2005), 1403–1413; and P. W. Kalivas and K. McFarland, "Brain circuitry and the reinstatement of cocaine-seeking behavior," *Psychopharmacology* 168 (2003), 44–56.

2. Linehan, "Emotion Regulation Handout #4," *DBT Skills Training Handouts and Worksheets*, 2nd ed. (New York: Guilford Press, 2014), 211; F. Lucantonio et al., "Transition from 'model-based' to 'model-free' behavioral control in addiction: involvement of the orbitofrontal cortex and dorsolateral striatum," *Neuropharmacology* 76, part B (January 2014), 407–415; C. B. Weng et al., "Gray matter and white matter abnormalities in online game addiction," *European Journal of Radiology* 82, no. 8 (2013), 1308–1312; and T. Hayashi, "Dorsolateral prefrontal and orbitofrontal cortex interactions during self-control of cigarette craving," *Proceedings of the National Academy of Sciences of the United States of America* 110, no. 11 (2013), 4422–4427.

3. C. P. O'Brien, "Anticraving medications for relapse prevention: a possible new class of psychoactive medications," *American Journal of Psychiatry* 162, no. 8 (August 2005), 1423–1431.

4. W. F. Velicer et al., "An empirical typology of subjects within stage of change," *Addictive Behaviors* 20, no. 3 (1995), 299–320; and J. O. Prochaska et al., "Stage-based expert systems to guide a population of primary care patients to quit smoking, eat healthier, prevent skin cancer, and receive regular mammograms," *Preventive Medicine* 41 (2005), 406–416.

5. K. N. Flegal, "Prevalence of obesity and trends in the distribution of body mass index among US adults, 1999-2010," *Journal of the American Medical Association* 307, no. 5 (2012), 491–497; and J. A. Colbert and S. Jangi, "Training physicians to manage obesity—back to the drawing board," *New England Journal of Medicine* 369, no. 15 (2013), 1389–1391.

6. R. C. Lawrence et al., "Estimates of the prevalence of arthritis and other rheumatic conditions in the United States. Part II," *Arthritis and Rheumatism* 58, no. 1 (2008), 26–35; S. P. Messier et al., "Effects of intensive diet and exercise on knee joint loads, inflammation, and clinical outcomes among overweight and obese adults with knee osteoarthritis: the IDEA randomized clinicial trial," *Journal of the American Medical Association* 310, no. 12 (2013), 1236–1273; K. Karason et al., "Heart rate variability in obesity and the effect of weight loss," *American Journal of Cardiology* 83, no. 8 (1999), 1242–1247; and H. S. Abed et al., "Effect of weight reduction and cardiometabolic risk factor management on symptom burden and severity in patients with atrial fibrillation: a randomized clinical trial," *Journal of the American Medical Association* 310, no. 19 (2013), 250–260.

7. A. E. Field et al., "The merits of subtyping obesity: one size does not fit all," *Journal of the American Medical Association* 310, no. 20 (2013), 2147–2148.

8. J. K. Elmquist et al., "Identifying hypothalamic pathways controlling food intake, body weight, and glucose homeostasis," *Journal of Comparative Neurology* 493 (2005), 63–71; S. Fulton et al., "Leptin regulation of the mesoaccumbens dopamine pathway," *Neuron* 51 (2006), 811–822; and J. C. Halford and J. E. Blundell, "Pharmacology of appetite suppression," *Progress in Drug Research* 54 (2000), 25–58.

9. J. D. Birkmeyer et al., "Surgical skill and complication rates after bariatric surgery," *New England Journal of Medicine* 369, no. 15 (October 10, 2013), 1434–1442; and A. P. Courcoulas et al., "Weight change and health outcomes at 3 years after bariatric surgery among individuals with severe obesity," *Journal of the American Medical Association* 310, no. 22 (2013), 2416–2425.

10. Elmquist et al., "Identifying hypothalamic pathways controlling food intake, body weight, and glucose homeostasis"; Fulton et al., "Leptin regulation of the mesoaccumbens dopamine pathway"; and Halford and Blundell, "Pharmacology of appetite suppression."

11. S. Zipfel et al., "Focal psychodynamic therapy, cognitive behaviour therapy, and optimised treatment as usual in outpatients with anorexia nervosa (ANTOP study): randomised controlled trial," *Lancet* 383 (2014), 127–137.

12. M. Pantell et al., "Social isolation: a predictor of mortality comparable to traditional clinical risk factors," *American Journal of Public Health* 103, no. 11 (November 2013), 2056–2062; Coan et al., "Lending a hand: social regulation of the neural response to threat"; Barbara Bradley Hagerty, "People who possess this one thing enjoy much better health as they age, science shows,"

The Washington Post, May 17, 2016.

13. M. J. Ostacher et al., "Impact of substance use disorders on recovery from episodes of depression in bipolar disorder patients: prospective data from the Systematic Treatment Enhancement Program for Bipolar Disorder (STEP-BD)," *American Journal of Psychiatry* 167 (2010), 289–297.

14. H. M Pettinati, "A double-blind, placebo-controlled trial combining sertraline and naltrexone for treating co-occurring depression and alcohol dependence," *American Journal of Psychiatry* 167 (2010), 668–675.

15. A. Torvik et al., "Brain lesions in alcoholics: a neuropathological study with clinical correlations," *Journal of the Neurological Sciences* 56 (1982), 233–248.

16. M. Huntgeburth et al., "Alcohol consumption and hypertension," *Current Hypertension Reports* 7 (2005), 180–185; and R. Providencia, "Cardiovascular protection from alcoholic drinks: scientific basis of the French paradox," *Revista Portuguesa de Cardiologia* 25 (2006), 1043–1058.

17. E. B. Foa, "Concurrent naltrexone and prolonged exposure therapy for patients with comorbid alcohol dependence and PTSD: a randomized clinical trial," *Journal of the American Medical Association* 310 (2013), 488–495.

18. T. B. Moyers, "From in-session behaviors to drinking outcomes: a causal chain for motivational interviewing," *Journal of Consulting and Clinical Psychology* 77 (2009), 1113–1124.

19. M. Bühler et al., "Nicotine dependence is characterized by disordered reward processing in a network driving motivation," *Biological Psychiatry* 67 (2010), 745–752; and E. J. Rose et al., "Acute nicotine differentially impacts anticipatory valence- and magnitude-related striatal activity," *Biological Psychiatry* 73 (2013), 280–288.

20. A. P. Groenman et al., "Stimulant treatment for attention-deficit hyperactivity disorder and risk of developing substance use disorder," *British Journal of Psychiatry* 203 (2013), 122–119.

21. M. E. Piper et al., "A randomized placebo-controlled clinical trial of five smoking cessation pharmacotherapies," *Archives of General Psychiatry* 66 (2009), 1253–1262.

22. R. N. Jamison et al., "Substance misuse treatment for high-risk chronic pain patients on opioid therapy: a randomized trial," *Pain* 150 (2010), 390–400.

23. C. L. Dodrill et al., "Prescription pain medication dependence," *American Journal of Psychiatry* 168 (2011), 466–471.

CHAPTER 4: BRAIN AND LEARNING STYLES

1. Lynda J. Katz, Gerald Goldstein, and Sue R. Beers, *Learning Disabilities in Older Adolescents and Adults: Clinical Utility of the Neuropsychological Perspective* (New York: Springer, 2001).

2. Jeffrey W. Gilger and Bonnie J. Kaplan, "The Concept of Atypical Brain Development (ABD) as Applied to Developmental Learning Disorders," chapter 3 in *Adult Learning Disorders: Contemporary Issues*, ed. Lorraine E. Wolf et al. (New York: Psychology Press, 2006), 57.

3. R. A. Brumback, "Warren A. Weinberg: pioneer in the field of learning disabilities," *Journal of Child Neurology* 19 (2004), 737.

4. Bryan Kolb and Ian Q. Whishaw, *Fundamentals of Human Neuropsychology*, 4th ed. (New York: W. H. Freeman, 1996).

5. N. Geschwind and A. M. Galaburda, "Cerebral lateralization: biological mechanisms, associations, and pathology. I: A hypothesis and a program for research," *Archives of Neurology* 42 (1985), 428–459.

6. A. Bechera, H. Damasio, D. Tranel, and A. R. Damasio, "Deciding advantageously before knowing the advantageous strategy," *Science* 275, no. 5304 (February 28, 1997), 1293–1295; and G. Vogel, "Scientists probe feelings behind decision-making," *Science* 275, no. 5304 (February 28, 1997), 1269.

7. Lee Ashendorf, Rod Swenson, and David J. Libon, eds., *The Boston Process Approach to Neuropsychological Assessment: A Practitioner's Guide* (New York: Oxford University Press, 2013).

8. J. J. McGough and R. A. Barkley, "Diagnostic controversies in adult attention deficit hyperactivity disorder," *American Journal of Psychiatry* 161 (2004), 1948–1956; and J. N. Giedd, A. C. Vaituzis, et al., "Quantitative MRI of the temporal lobe, amygdala, and hippocampus in normal human development: ages 4-18," *Journal of Comparative Neurology* 366 (1996), 223–230.

9. B. A. Shaywitz, G. R. Lyon, and S. E. Shaywitz, "The role of functional magnetic resonance imaging in understanding reading and dyslexia," *Developmental Neuropsychology* 30 (2006), 613–632.

10. S. Birch and C. Chase, "Visual and language processing deficits in compensated and uncompensated college students with dyslexia," *Journal of Learning Disabilities* 37 (2004), 389–410; M. Wolf and P. G. Bowers, "The double-deficit hypothesis for the developmental dyslexias," *Journal of Educational Psychology* 91 (1999), 415–438; G. F. Eden et al., "Neural changes following remediation in adult developmental dyslexia," *Neuron* 44 (2004), 411–422; S. E. Shaywitz, "Persistence of dyslexia: the Connecticut Longitudinal Study at adolescence," *Pediatrics* 104 (1999), 1351–1359; and A. M. Galaburda et al., "Developmental dyslexia: four consecutive patients with cortical abnormalities," *Annals of Neurology* 18 (1985), 222–233.

11. Jack M. Fletcher, G. Reid Lyon, Lynn S. Fuchs, and Marcia A. Barnes, *Learning Disabilities: From Identification to Intervention* (New York: Guilford Press, 2007).

12. B. A. Shaywitz, et al., "Sex differences in the functional organization of the brain for language," *Nature* 373 (1995), 607–609; A. S. Clark et al., "Androgen binding and metabolism in the cerebral cortex of the developing rhesus monkey," *Endocrinology* 123 (1988), 932–940; J. K. Morse et al., "Gonadal steroids influence axon sprouting in the hippocampal dentate gyrus: a sexually dimorphic response," *Experimental Neurology* 94 (1986), 649–658; Kathryn Kniele and Ruben C. Gur, "Sex Differences in Brain Development and Learning Disability," chapter 2 in *Adult Learning Disorders: Contemporary Issues*, ed. Lorraine E. Wolf et al. (New York: Psychology Press, 2006), 29; M. L. Kalbfleisch, "Functional neuroanatomy of talent," *The Anatomical Record* Part B, 277 (2004), 21–36; and N. Geschwind and A. M. Galaburda, *Cerebral*

Lateralization: Biological Mechanisms, Associations, and Pathology (MIT Press: Cambridge, MA, 1987).

13. Simon Baron-Cohen, *The Science of Evil: On Empathy and the Origins of Cruelty* (New York: Basic Books, 2011); Aaron T. Beck, Denise D. Davis, and Arthur Freeman, eds., *Cognitive Therapy of Personality Disorders*, 3rd edition (New York: Guilford Press: 2014); John J. Ratey and Catherine Johnson, "The Biology of Being 'Difficult,'" chapter 2 in *Shadow Syndromes* (New York: Pantheon Books, 1997), 66-99; Marsha M. Linehan, "Dialectical behavioral therapy: a cognitive behavioral approach to parasuicide," *Journal of Personality Disorders* 1, no. 4 (1987), 328–333; and Marsha M. Linehan, "Dialectical behavioral therapy for borderline personality disorder. Theory and method," *Bulletin of the Menninger Clinic* 51 (1987), 261–276.

14. Linehan, *DBT Skills Training Handouts and Worksheets*, 341–352.

Chapter 5: Memory

1. A. R. Damasio, "The brain binds entities and events by multiregional activation from convergence zones," *Neural Computation* 1 (1989), 123–132; J. L. McClelland, "Constructive Memory and Memory Distortions: A Parallel-Distributed Processing Approach," in *Memory Distortion*, ed. D. L. Schacter (Cambridge, MA: Harvard University Press, 1995), 69–90; J. V. Haxby, et al., "Distributed Hierarchical Neural Systems for Visual Memory in Human Cortex," in *Connections, Cognition, and Alzheimer's Disease*, ed. B. T. Hyman et al. (Berlin: Springer-Verlag, 1997), 167– 180; and M. Seeck et al., "Selectively distributed processing of visual object recognition in the temporal and frontal lobes of the human brain," *Annals of Neurology* 37 (1995), 538–545.

2. L. I. Benowitz et al., "Localization of the growth-associated phosphoprotein GAP-43 (B-50, F1) in the human cerebral cortex," *Journal of Neuroscience* 9 (1989), 990–995; and T. V. Bliss and G. L. Collingridge, "A synaptic model of memory: long-term potentiation in the hippocampus," *Nature* 361 (1993), 31–39.

3. F. A. Wilson and E. T. Rolls, "Neuronal responses related to the novelty and familiarity of visual stimuli in the substantia innominata, diagonal band of Broca and periventricular region of the primate basal forebrain," *Experimental Brain Research* 80 (1990), 104–120; D. R. Britton et al., "Brain norepinephrine depleting lesions selectively enhance behavioral responsiveness to novelty," *Physiology & Behavior* 33 (1984), 473–478; E. M. Pich et al., "Common neural substrates for the addictive properties of nicotine and cocaine," *Science* 275, no. 5296 (1997), 83–86; M. J. Lewis, "Alcohol reinforcement and neuropharmacological therapeutics," *Alcohol and Alcoholism* 31, suppl 1 (1996), 17–25; and P. D. Wall and G. D. Davis, "Three cerebral cortical systems affecting autonomic function," *Journal of Neurophysiology* 14 (1951), 507–517.

4. M. M. Mesulam, *Principles of Behavioral and Cognitive Neurology*, 2nd ed. (New York: Oxford University Press, 2000), 30.

5. Ibid., 441.

6. S. Weintraub et al., "Successful cognitive aging: individual differences among physicians on a computerized test of mental state," *Journal of Geriatric Psy-*

chiatry 27, no. 1 (1994), 15–34; and J. D. Williams and M. G. Klug, "Aging and cognition: methodological differences in outcome," *Experimental Aging Research* 22, no. 3 (1996), 219–244.

7. C. Geula and M. M. Mesulam, "Cholinergic Systems and Related Neuropathological Predilection Patterns in Alzheimer's Disease," in *Alzheimer's Disease*, ed. R. D. Terry et al. (New York: Raven Press, 1994) 263–291; and E. Masliah et al., "Quantitative synaptic alterations in the human neocortex during normal aging," *Neurology* 43 (1993), 192–197.

8. Mesulam, *Principles of Behavioral and Cognitive Neurology*, 442.

9. E. E. Devore et al., "Sleep duration in midlife and later life in relation to cognition," *Journal of the American Geriatrics Society* 62, no. 6 (2014), 1073–1081.

10. L. K. Lee et al., "Docosahexaenoic acid-concentrated fish oil supplementation in subjects with mild cognitive impairment (MCI): a 12-month randomised, double-blind, placebo-controlled trial," *Psychopharmacology* 225 (2013), 605–612.

11. G. Douaud et al., "Preventing Alzheimer's disease-related gray matter atrophy by B-vitamin treatment," *Proceedings of the National Academy of Sciences of the United States of America* 110 (2013), 9523–9528.

12. D. Wade, "Applying the WHO ICF framework to the rehabilitation of patients with cognitive deficits," in *The Effectiveness of Rehabilitation for Cognitive Deficits*, ed. P. Halligan and D. Wade (Oxford: Oxford University Press, 2013), 421; and M. G. Gelder et al. eds, *New Oxford Textbook of Psychiatry*, 2nd edition (Oxford: Oxford University Press, 2012).

13. D. H. Daneshvar, et al., "The epidemiology of sport-related concussion," *Clinical Sports Medicine* 30, no. 1 (2011), 1–17.

14. W. A. Lishman, "Brain damage in relation to psychiatric disability after head injury," *British Journal of Psychiatry* 114 (1968), 373–410; and C. Symonds, "Concussion and its sequelae," *The Lancet* 1 (1962), 1–5.

15. J. J. Bazarian et al., "Diffusion tensor imaging detects clinically important axonal damage after mild traumatic brain injury: a pilot study," *Journal of Neurotrauma* 24 (2007), 1447–59; M. X. Huang et al., "Integrated imaging approach with MEG and DTI to detect mild traumatic brain injury in military and civilian patients," *Journal of Neurotrauma* 26 (2009), 1213–26; and S. N. Niogi et al., "Extent of microstructural white matter injury in post-concussive syndrome correlates with impaired cognitive reaction time: a 3T diffusion tensor imaging study of mild traumatic brain injury," *American Journal of Neuroradiology* 29 (2008), 967–73.

16. A. Al Sayegh et al., "Psychological approaches to treatment of postconcussion syndrome: a systematic review," *Journal of Neurology, Neurosurgery, and Psychiatry* 81 (2010), 1128–34.

17. S. J. Mitchell and M. H. Bennett, "Unestablished indications for hyperbaric oxygen therapy," *Diving and Hyperbaric Medicine Journal* 44, no. 4 (2014), 228–34; and confidential personal communication (study in progress).

18. M. R. Lamprecht and B. Morrison, "A combination therapy of 17-beta-estradiol and memantine is more neuroprotective than monotherapies in an organotypic

brain slice culture model of traumatic brain injury," *Journal of Neurotrauma* 32, no. 17 (2015), 1361–1368.

19. H. M. Francis et al., "Reduced heart rate variability in chronic severe traumatic brain injury: association with impaired emotional and social functioning, and potential for treatment using biofeedback," *Neuropsychological Rehabilitation* 26, no. 1 (2016), 103–125.

20. M. A. Naeser et al., "Significant improvements in cognitive performance post-transcranial, red/near-infrared light-emitting diode treatments in chronic, mild traumatic brain injury: open protocol study," *Journal of Neurotrauma* 31, no. 11 (2014), 1008–1017.

21. R. Sullivan et al., "A possible new focus for stroke treatment: migrating stem cells," *Expert Opinion on Biological Therapy* 15 (2015), 1–10; and A. Sharma et al., "Cell therapy attempted as a novel approach for chronic traumatic brain injury: a pilot study," *SpringerPlus* 4, no. 26 (2015).

22. S. K. Lakkaraju et al., "Cyclopropyl-containing positive allosteric modulators of metabotropic glutamate receptor subtype 5," *Bioorganic and Medicinal Chemistry Letters* 25, no. 11 (2015), 2275–2279.

23. W. Y. Ong et al., "Synthetic and natural inhibitors of phospholipases A2: their importance for understanding and treatment of neurological disorders," *ACS Chemical Neuroscience* 6, no. 6 (2015), 814–831.

24. J. C. Morris, "The clinical dementia rating scale (CDR): current vision and scoring rules," *Neurology* 43 (1993), 2412–2414.

25. E. Levy-Lahad and T. D. Bird, "Genetic factors in Alzheimer's disease: a review of recent advances," *Annals of Neurology* 40 (1996), 829–840; J. Hardy, "Amyloid, the presenilins and Alzheimer's disease," *Trends in Neurosciences* 20 (1997), 154–159; E. Storey et al., "Alzheimer's disease amyloid precursor protein on the surface of cortical neurons in primary culture co-localizes with adhesion patch components," *Brain Research* 735 (1996), 217–231; and D. A. Evans et al., "Prevalence of Alzheimer's disease in a community population of older persons: higher than previously reported," *Journal of the American Medical Association* 262 (1989), 2551–2556.

26. M. A. Pericak-Vance et al., "Complete genomic screen in late-onset familial Alzheimer disease: evidence for a new locus on chromosome 12," *Journal of the American Medical Association* 278, no. 15 (1997), 1237–1241; A. D. Roses, "The predictive value of APOE genotyping in the early diagnosis of dementia of the Alzheimer's type: data from three independent series," K. Iqbel et al., eds., *Alzheimer's Disease: Biology, Diagnosis and Therapeutics* (West Sussex, England: John Wiley & Sons, 1997), 85–91; and J. C. Morris et al., "Cerebral amyloid deposition and diffuse plaques in 'normal' aging: evidence for presymptomatic and very mild Alzheimer's disease," *Neurology* 46 (1996), 707–719.

27. L. Xu et al., "Behavioural stress facilitates the induction of long-term depression in the hippocampus," *Nature* 387 (1997), 497–500; and D. M. Diamond and G. M. Rose, "Stress impairs LTP and hippocampal-dependent memory," *Annals of the New York Academy of Sciences* 746 (1994), 411–414.

CHAPTER 6: BODY, MIND, BRAIN

1. Beck, Davis, and Freeman, eds., *Cognitive Therapy of Personality Disorders.*

2. P. D. MacLean, "Psychosomatic disease and the visceral brain: recent developments bearing on the Papez theory of emotion," *Psychosomatic Medicine* 11 (1949), 338–353; and Q. Aziz et al., "Identification of human brain loci processing esophageal sensation using positron emission tomography," *Gastroenterology* 113 (1997), 50–59.

3. M. M. Mesulam and E. J. Mufson, "Insula of the old world monkey. III: efferent cortical output and comments on function," *Journal of Comparative Neurology* 212 (1982), 38–52; B. R. Kaada, K. H. Pribram, and J. A. Epstein, "Respiratory and vascular responses in monkeys from temporal pole, insula, orbital surface and cingulate gyrus: a preliminary report," *Journal of Neurophysiology* 12 (1949), 347–356; W. Penfield and M. E. Faulk, "The insula: further observations on its function," *Brain* 78 (1955), 445–470; B. L. Hoffman and T. Rasmussen, "Stimulation studies of insular cortex of *macaca mulatta*," *Journal of Neurophysiology* 16 (1953), 343–351; M. J. Showers and E. W. Lauer, "Somatovisceral motor patterns in the insula," *Journal of Comparative Neurology* 117 (1961), 107–115; M. Hadjivassiliou et al., "Does cryptic gluten sensitivity play a part in neurological illness?" *The Lancet* 347 (1996), 369–371; M. Hadjivassiliou et al., "Clinical, radiological, neurophysiological, and neuropathological characteristics of gluten ataxia," *The Lancet* 352 (1998), 1582–1585; J. S. Trier, "Celiac sprue and refractory sprue," in *Gastrointestinal and Liver Disease: Pathophysiology/Diagnosis/Management*, 6th edition, ed. M. Feldman et al. (Philadelphia: W. B. Saunders, 1998), 1557–1573; P. F. Chinnery et al., "CSF antigliadin antibodies and the Ramsay Hunt syndrome," *Neurology* 49 (1997), 1131–1133; G. Gobbi et al., "Coeliac disease, epilepsy, and cerebral calcifications," *The Lancet* 340 (1992), 439–443; and A. Fasano and A. Catassi, "Current approaches to diagnosis and treatment of celiac disease: an evolving spectrum," *Gastroenterology* 120 (2001), 636–651.

4. E. J. Dropcho, "Remote neurological manifestations of cancer," *Neurologic Clinics* 20, no. 1 (2002), 85–122.

5. J. Reiher et al., "Temporal intermittent rhythmic delta activity (TIRDA) in the diagnosis of complex partial epilepsy: sensitivity, specificity, and predictive value," *Canadian Journal of Neurological Sciences* 16 (1989), 398–401.

INDEX

with potential and purpose,
206–208
problems, *280*
AIDS, *280*
Alcoholism, *280. See also* Addiction,
alcohol
Alcohol, memory and, 192
Allergies
addiction and, 120, 121
anxiety and, 51, 59, 68
brain, learning styles and, 167, 169,
170, 181
depression and, 27
hay fever, *298*
intuitive readings and, xx, 12
medicines for, 191, 193
mood, immune disorders and, 249,
252–253
problems/causes/new thought pattern, *280, 298*
*All Is Well: Heal Your Body with Medicine,
Affirmations, and Intuition* (Hay and
Schulz), xxi, 254, 265
Alzheimer's disease, *280*
about: effects on brain and what it
is, 188, 201, 228
acetylcholine and, 191
brain changes associated with,
233–235
brain fog and, 43
hope for other dementias and. *See*
Memory disorders, Alzheimer's
and other dementias
menopause and, 199–200
normal aging and, 201–202
Susan's story (Do I have Alzheimer's?). *See* Memory, depression
impacting
Amenorrhea, *280*
Amino acids, 156
Amnesia, *280*
Amygdala
fear, anxiety and, 49, 53–55, 56, 60
functions of, 49
intuition and, 49
memory and, 188–189, 208, 213
as one type of memory (body memory), 56, 188–189, 208. *See also*
Hippocampus
rewiring brain and, 82–83

Amyotrophic Lateral Sclerosis (ALS, or
Lou Gehrig's Dis-ease), *280*
Anemia, 12, 124, 201, *280*
Anger
becoming medical (steps delineated),
4–7
biochemistry of, 4–7
brain relationships, 8
defined, 3, 7–8
sadness and, mind-body network,
7–9
stopping before affects health, 3–4
Ankle(s), 108, *281*
Anorectal bleeding, *281*
Anorexia, *281. See also* Addiction, to
being thin; Eating disorders
Antidepressants, 7, 13, 18–20, 32, 33,
63, 64, 75
Anus, issues with, *281. See also* Hemorrhoids
Anxiety, 47–90, *281. See also* Fear; *specific types immediately following*
about: overview of, 47
brain-body, 48–49
emotional centers associations,
50–52
emotional symptoms indicating
physical issues, 241–244
hormones and. *See* Hormones, heart
issues, and brain
medical intuition and, 49–52
medicines and supplements for, 61
memory and. *See* Memory, anxiety,
trauma and
spiritual experiences and. *See* Spiritual orientation and illumination
Anxiety, chronic worry, 58–67
Adele's story, 59–67
affirmations, 64–67
body symptoms, 58–59
facts from intuitive reading, 60
intuitive reading, 59
medicines and supplements for,
63–64
mind symptoms, 58
solution, 60–61
treatments, 61
Anxiety, obsessive and compulsive,
67–72
affirmations, 72

anxiety and, 85
body, mind, brain and, 243, 262
brain fog and, 43
depression and, 5, 6
fourth center and, xviii, xx, 13
hormones, brain and, 255–256
hormone therapy and, 261
memory and, 228
tests for, 261–262
Hematochezia, *281*
Hemorrhoids, *298*
Hepatitis, *298*
Hernia, *299*
Herpes, 228, *299*
Hetty's story, 36–40
Hippocampus
aging, memory and, 201–202, 206–207
changing over time, 56
memory and, 188–189, 199–200
menopause, memory and, 199–200
as one type of memory (mind memory), 56, 188–189, 208. *See also* Amygdala
plaques, tangles in, 201
rewiring brain and, 82–83
sleep importance for, 156
trauma, brain circuits and, 56, 208
Hip(s)/hip problems, xviii, *294, 299*
Hirsutism, *299*
Hives, *299*
Hobbies, 62–63
Hodgkin's dis-ease, *299*
Holding fluids, *300*
Hormone replacement, 31–32, 251, 260–261
Hormones, heart issues, and brain, 255–262. *See also* Menopause and perimenopause; Testopause
Abigail's story (paralyzed by anxiety), 250–256
adrenal gland, mood and, 251–252. *See also* Adrenal gland
Blanche's story (hormonal anxiety), 257–262
body symptoms, 250–251, 257
facts from intuitive readings, 251, 257–258
immune disorders, mood and, 252–253

intuitive readings, 250, 257
signs of imbalances, 255–256
solutions, 253–254, 258–259, 262
your medical intuitive reading, 259–262
Hormones, stabilizing brain-body, 30–31
Horney, Karen, 8
Huntington's dis-ease, *300*
Hyperactivity, *300. See also* Attention deficit hyperactivity disorder (ADHD)
Hyperbaric oxygen, 191–192, 224, 226, 237
Hyperthyroidism, 78, *300*
Hyperventilation, *300*
Hypoglycemia, 201, *300*
Hypothyroidism, 13, 51, 59, *300*

I

Ileitis, *300*
Immune system disorders
adrenal function, brain and, 249–251
medical intuition and, 254
mood and, 252–253
parasites, infections and, 229
rewiring memory/thoughts between mind/body, 254–255
symptoms, 249–250
Impotence, 51, *300*
Incontinence, *301*
Incurable, *301*
Indigestion, *301*
Infections, xx, 15, 27, 42, 229, *301. See also* Immune system disorders; Viral infections
Inflammation, *301*
brain fog and, 20
dementia and, 6
depression and, 5, 6, 17–18, 19, 21, 30
emotions causing, 247–248
immune disorders, mood and, 252–253, 256
medicines affecting, 19
memory and, 192–193, 203, 206, 221, 222, 223, 225, 226, 228, 235
reducing, 206, 222, 223, 225, 235, 237, *301, 302*
stress, cytokines and, 5, 12
weight and, 108

ADHD and, 155–156
  affirmation, 131
  alcohol consumption and, 124, 125, 126, 127
  anxiety and, 58, 80
  depression and, 5, 6, 11, 15, 41
  herbs for, 213
  magnesium for, 80, 213
  memory and, 191, 193–194, 203
  pills for, side effects, 191
Sleep apnea, 43
Smoking, 135–136, 154, 158, 266. *See also* Addictions, multiple
Snoring, *314*
Solar plexus, *314*
Sores, *314. See also* Canker sores; Cold sores (fever blisters)
Sore throat, *314*
Spasms, *314*
Spastic colitis, *314*
Spinal meningitis, *314*
Spine, *314. See also* Back problems
Spine, curvature of (scoliosis), 82, *312*, *314*
Spiritual journeys, 44
Spiritual orientation and illumination. *See also* Wholeness
  affirmations, 272
  body, mind, brain and, 267–273
  body symptoms, 269
  brain fog and, 43
  brain structure, balance and, 176–177
  Denise's story (mystical brain), 268–273
  emotional/physical health problems and, 267
  facts from intuitive reading, 269–270
  intuitive reading, 268–269
  seizures and, 271
  solution, 270–272
  transformation of brain and body, 267–273
Spleen, *314*
Sprains, *315*
Sterility, *315*
Sties, *315*
Stiff neck, *315*
Stomach and stomach problems, *315*

Stress. *See also* Cortisol
  meditation for. *See* Meditation
  reducing, for memory, 236
  switching brain from fear to safety, 56–57
Stroke, *315*
Stuttering, *315*
Suicide, *315*
Superiority. *See* Right brain learning disorders
Supplements. *See* Medicines and supplements; *specific medicines and supplements*
Swelling, *315. See also* Edema; Fluids, holding; Inflammation
Syphilis, *316*

T

Tapeworm, *316*
Teeth and teeth problems, *316*, *318*, *319. See also* Root canal
Temporal lobe
  addiction and, 141
  ADHD, focusing and, 153
  anger associated with, 8
  balance of frontal lobe and, 38, 175–176, 177–179
  functions of, 7, 271
  mystical brain and, 271–272
  personality and, 175–179, 217
Temporomandibular joint (TMJ) syndrome, *302*
Terry's story (trauma and memory), 211–215
Testicles, *316*
Testopause, 255, 258, 260–261
Testosterone, 27, 43, 146, 224, 242, 256, 258–259, 261
Tetanus (lockjaw), *303*, *316*
Third center, xviii, xx, 12, 51, 95–96, 99–100, 102, 110, 119, 148, 189, 236–237
Thoughts, forming experiences, xv
Throat and throat problems, *314*, *316*
Thrush, *317*
Thymus, *317*
Thyroid. *See also* Fifth center
  addiction and, 117, 119, 126
  anxiety and, 51, 59, 78

ACKNOWLEDGMENTS

This book is about how we can heal our minds and create wholeness. We are not an island unto ourselves; everyone has a unique genius, and also some weakness in the brain as well. So none of us truly has a "complete" brain. To sail through life, be healthy, happy, and productive, we have to hire, marry, or befriend people who provide the parts of the brain we don't have. I am grateful for all the help I receive daily from people who give me their excellence, their genius. So brace yourself. Here's the list. I've arranged them by brain areas for the obvious reason.

The Frontal Lobe Executive Area

Louise Hay, Executive-in-Chief. She is the great legend in mind-body medicine. Whether on Skype going over case studies or through her lectures and books, she is an unsung hero of psychiatry and cognitive behavioral therapy. I spent 35 years educating myself, trying to put together, bit by bit, a connection between emotion, intuition, the brain, body, and health. However, she sat in a room listening to clients' stories and came up with the same information. Go figure. I'm honored to be with and work with this giant of a woman.

Running the organization of Hay House for planning, problem solving, and forward thinking, thank you to Hay House CEO Reid Tracy and COO Margarete Nielsen, who continue to give me fantastic opportunities. Patty Gift, Vice President–Editorial, a legend in this industry, I bow to you with respect, admiration, and love. For decision-making skills and publicity, Lindsay McGinty, thank you for handling my "social phobia." Many thanks to Marlene Robinson, who is invaluable in her attention to endorsements, and to Christy Salinas, for the book cover. Pantone colors, who knew? I am thrilled Laura Gray does my online courses. She is so organized, she could probably write her own book. For the machine that skillfully moves those great "I can do it!" Hay House conferences across the United States, thank you for giving me yearly gigs.

THE LEFT BRAIN

Anne Barthel, my trusted editor. She's translated my words so they sound coherent. You capture my Boston, Rhode Island, and pseudo-New York accents. How do you do it? I submitted your name to the Vatican for sainthood. Ditto to my transcriptionist, Karen Kinne. How could I live without you? You type the voice in my head.

Thank you to Kripalu and Susie "Debbie" Arnett. You monitor and direct my career in a way that is impossible to describe. Whether it's conferences or TV production, you help broadcast my career. And while we're on broadcasting, thanks go to Hay House Radio. You rock, and you rock hard! Diane Ray, Richelle, and all the crew. Every week for over 10 years you are there so I can say, "Intuitive Health with Dr. Mona Lisa. Can I take the next caller?"

Moving on to the brain's learning and memory areas. The following people have taught me about the brain and its connections to the body. Thank you to my past mentors. Every moment with these people made a contribution in this book. Dr. Margaret Naeser; M. Marcel Mesulam, M.D.; Deepak Pandya, M.D.; Edith Kaplan, Ph.D.; Norman Geschwind, M.D.; Christiane Northrup, M.D.; and Joan Borysenko, Ph.D.

THE RIGHT BRAIN

On a neuropsychological evaluation, I have what we would call a double-A frontal lobe, which is why the lengthy list of support above and below. My weaker left hemisphere requires the genius of my editor. I do have a double-D right brain, thank God, so now I thank the divine for having given me those abilities I do have, to receive the information and create this book. Without God, I am nothing. Really. I would not be alive without your help. Literally.

THE BODY

We wouldn't have a complete mind if our brain wasn't grounded by our body. These individuals are a loving foundation, my family. They help me sail forward and maybe even saunter through daily life. As a medical intuitive, of course, I will organize their names in terms of emotional centers, or energy centers, if you prefer.

7th Center: Helping me hold a spiritual connection, Avis Smith is a rare Hebrew teacher and Torah scholar. I am proud to call her my chavrusa. To the staff of Disney World, Magic Kingdom, Epcot, Animal Kingdom, and Hollywood Studios: Thank you for not filing a restraining order due to the excessive number of visits I have made to maintain my sanity in the last year. BTW, I will be renewing my yearly membership once again.

6th Center: Colleagues and friends. Thank you to Gypsy Hands with Sarah Xochitl Griscom, Jessica, and staff. These Knoxville Healers, they are the jelly to my peanut butter. Daniel Peralta, a scamp and fellow Gucci aficionado. How can you not love Daniel? Heather Dane, whose mind has an encyclopedic knowledge of nutrition. You should taste her wheat-free, dairy-free Samoas!

5th Center: My voice. To Jay Hoffman and Marshall Bellovin, thank you for expert, balanced, legal advice. You are my Perry Masons. Merci to website master Jeffrey Sutherland, who has remarkably stable blood pressure in the midst of sometimes stressful Internet glitches.

<u>4th Center</u>: For people who have kept my heart beating and health stable. Dr. Kumar Kakarla, Dr. Rosemary Duda, Dr. Fern Tsao, Dr. Dean Deng, Dr. Steven Dobieski, and Mayo Clinic. I bow to you, you are amazing! Thank you, Anthem Blue Cross and Blue Shield for paying the bills!

<u>3rd Center</u>: Appearance. Let's start with the hair, which is always a deal. To Akari Studios, Peter John (the cut) and Jeffrey (the color). Thank you! To the wonderful Mike Brewer. He keeps the lawns, gardens, and my holiday inflatables inflated. To Heather and Anita at QCS. My house has never been cleaner. Food, banquet, and conferences: Food could be an issue, but it's not if I go to the Harraseeket Inn in Freeport, Maine. They keep me alive with organic food. Thank you to owners Rodney, Chip Gray, Nancy Gray, barkeeper Ronda Real, chef MaryAnn McAllister, manager Marsha, Jeanne-Marie, banquets, and all the waitstaff. If any of you readers are lucky enough to go there, get the gluten-free apple and blueberry pie. Say I sent you, but don't take my seat at the bar!

<u>2nd Center</u>: The money. Thank you to my money team— George Howard, Paul Chabot, and Peter, the accountant. They hold the reins when I have lost mine.

<u>1st Center</u>: I am extremely grateful to have the most amazing friends and family. When you people listed read this, don't get upset at the order. It's impossible to make all of you first, so I've made you hyphenated in one sentence. Caroline Myss–Janie and Jerry LeMole–Naomi Judd–Larry Strickland–Helen and Roy Snow–Laura Day–Joyce Bowers. The hyphenated list makes you one big whole family in my life, all of whom I love you to pieces. But let me express my thanks, in detail, in reverse alphabetical order.

Caroline Myss, my conjoined twin, separated at birth and put up for adoption. We have cried and laughed on the phone. We share the Autosomal Dominant gene for Mont Blanc pens, animated art, and several biological conditions that are too numerous to list. You make me feel so loved. Oh, what would the world be like without you?

To Drs. Janie and Gerald LeMole for being there in Phoenix, Arizona, when I, as they say, almost bought the farm. You saved my life, helped me walk again. Thank you!

Miss Naomi and Mr. Larry, assorted canines, everyone else around Peaceful Valley; Helen and Roy Snow, and everyone in Leiper's Fork. You've prayed for me. We've laughed, cried, through floods, car crashes, national disasters. All the good times with a southern drawl, you've said, "Well, honey, we lo-ove you!"

Laura Day, my Sephardic-sister, although she denies she is this. A relationship via texts, e-mails, phone calls in her apartment in New York City. I love you more than my luggage, and that takes some.

To my southeast Florida family—the Bowers Family, especially to Joyce Bowers, who makes me laugh with her New York accent and attitude all packed into her five-foot-eleven height. She reminds me of Judge Judy, who, as everyone knows, I've watched faithfully for 20 years. You push me, push me to be better and restrain me when I'm going astray. Thank you.

To my precious babies, Loretta Lynn, Conway Twitty, Tammy Wynette. Yes, that's a nod to the Southern influence. And of course, Horatio. I love you people.

And finally, I am so grateful to you, the reader. There would be no book if it weren't for you. Thank you for being there.

ABOUT THE AUTHORS

Dr. Mona Lisa Schulz is one of those rare people who can cross the borders of intuition, science, medicine, and mysticism. An internationally known expert in Medical Intuition and Mind-Body Medicine, she has authored and co-authored books published in 27 languages. With quick wit, accent, and style, and medical and scientific credentials, Dr. Mona Lisa intuitively pinpoints how specific health problems in our bodies can be solved by unraveling all the emotional, relationship, environmental, vocational, and spiritual issues in our lives. With her M.D., board certification in psychiatry, and Ph.D. in brain science, she's been the expert-on-intuition guest on *The Oprah Winfrey Show, CBS This Morning*, and Dr. Oz Radio, has hosted her own Hay House Radio program for over a decade, and has appeared on many other national and international TV and radio programs. Dr. Mona Lisa teaches individuals from around the world in her Annual Medical Intuition 7-Day Certificate Training Institute in Freeport, Maine. A medical intuitive for over 30 years and a practicing neuropsychiatrist, Dr. Mona Lisa has published five books, *Heal Your Mind* (with Louise Hay), *All Is Well* (with Louise Hay), *The Intuitive Advisor, The New Feminine Brain,* and *Awakening Intuition.* She lives between Yarmouth, Maine, Nashville, and Florida with her four cats and assorted wildlife.

Louise Hay, the author of the international bestseller *You Can Heal Your Life*, is a metaphysical lecturer and teacher with more than 50 million books sold worldwide. For more than 30 years, she has helped people throughout the world discover and implement the full potential of their own creative powers for personal growth and self-healing. She has appeared on *The Oprah Winfrey Show* and many other TV and radio programs both in the U.S. and abroad. Websites: www.LouiseHay.com® and www.HealYourLife.com®

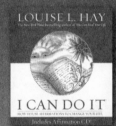
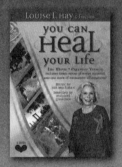
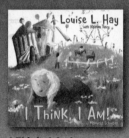

We hope you enjoyed this Hay House book. If you'd like
to receive our online catalog featuring additional information
on Hay House books and products, or if you'd like to find
out more about the Hay Foundation, please contact:

Hay House, Inc., P.O. Box 5100, Carlsbad, CA 92018-5100
(760) 431-7695 or (800) 654-5126
(760) 431-6948 (fax) or (800) 650-5115 (fax)
www.hayhouse.com® • www.hayfoundation.org

○ ○ ○

Published and distributed in Australia by: Hay House Australia
Pty. Ltd., 18/36 Ralph St., Alexandria NSW 2015 • *Phone:* 612-9669-4299
Fax: 612-9669-4144 • www.hayhouse.com.au

Published and distributed in the United Kingdom by: Hay House UK, Ltd.,
Astley House, 33 Notting Hill Gate, London W11 3JQ • *Phone:* 44-20-3675-2450
Fax: 44-20-3675-2451 • www.hayhouse.co.uk

Published and distributed in the Republic of South Africa by:
Hay House SA (Pty), Ltd., P.O. Box 990, Witkoppen 2068 • info@hayhouse.co.za
www.hayhouse.co.za

Published in India by: Hay House Publishers India, Muskaan Complex, Plot No.
3, B-2, Vasant Kunj, New Delhi 110 070 • *Phone:* 91-11-4176-1620
Fax: 91-11-4176-1630 • www.hayhouse.co.in

Distributed in Canada by: Raincoast Books, 2440 Viking Way,
Richmond, B.C. V6V 1N2 • *Phone:* 1-800-663-5714
Fax: 1-800-565-3770 • www.raincoast.com

○ ○ ○

Take Your Soul on a Vacation

Visit www.HealYourLife.com® to regroup, recharge,
and reconnect with your own magnificence.
Featuring blogs, mind-body-spirit news, and life-changing
wisdom from Louise Hay and friends.

Visit www.HealYourLife.com today!

Free e-newsletters from Hay House, the Ultimate Resource for Inspiration

Be the first to know about Hay House's dollar deals, free downloads, special offers, affirmation cards, giveaways, contests, and more!

 Get exclusive excerpts from our latest releases and videos from *Hay House Present Moments*.

 Enjoy uplifting personal stories, how-to articles, and healing advice, along with videos and empowering quotes, within *Heal Your Life*.

 Have an inspirational story to tell and a passion for writing? Sharpen your writing skills with insider tips from *Your Writing Life*.

Sign Up Now!

Get inspired, educate yourself, get a complimentary gift, and share the wisdom!

http://www.hayhouse.com/newsletters.php

Visit www.hayhouse.com to sign up today!

 HAY HOUSE

 HAYHOUSE RADIO
radio for your soul®

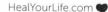 HealYourLife.com

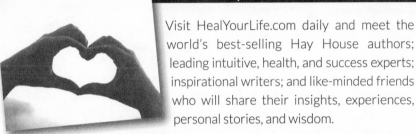
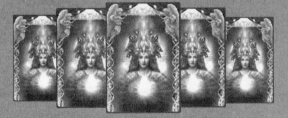